Higo José Neri da Silva
Kátia da Conceição Machado
Keylla da Conceição Machado

Updates in Pharmacology

AF570921

Higo José Neri da Silva
Kátia da Conceição Machado
Keylla da Conceição Machado

Updates in Pharmacology

Health articles

ScienciaScripts

Imprint

Any brand names and product names mentioned in this book are subject to trademark, brand or patent protection and are trademarks or registered trademarks of their respective holders. The use of brand names, product names, common names, trade names, product descriptions etc. even without a particular marking in this work is in no way to be construed to mean that such names may be regarded as unrestricted in respect of trademark and brand protection legislation and could thus be used by anyone.

Cover image: www.ingimage.com

This book is a translation from the original published under ISBN 978-620-6-76098-6.

Publisher:
Sciencia Scripts
is a trademark of
Dodo Books Indian Ocean Ltd. and OmniScriptum S.R.L publishing group

120 High Road, East Finchley, London, N2 9ED, United Kingdom
Str. Armeneasca 28/1, office 1, Chisinau MD-2012, Republic of Moldova, Europe
Printed at: see last page
ISBN: 978-620-8-01574-9

Copyright © Higo José Neri da Silva, Kátia da Conceição Machado, Keylla da Conceição Machado
Copyright © 2024 Dodo Books Indian Ocean Ltd. and OmniScriptum S.R.L publishing group

CHAPTER 1

ANTIBIOTIC CONTROL IN THE HOSPITAL PHARMACY: A SYSTEMATIC REVIEW

CONTROL OF ANTIBIOTICS IN HOSPITAL PHARMACY: A SYSTEMATIC REVIEW

ANTIBIOTIC CONTROL IN HOSPITAL PHARMACY: A SYSTEMATIC REVIEW

Manoela Carine Lima de Freitas Gustavo Mariano Duarte de Souza Evetrycyely Vieira de Sousa Tamara Rocha Silva Sousa

SUMMARY

In the 1980s, Brazil was marked by advances in the control of HIs, which began to raise the awareness of health professionals, where the first Hospital Infection Control Commissions emerged. The main objective of this study is to evaluate publications on antibiotic control in hospital pharmacies. Data was collected from the following scientific databases: Latin American and Caribbean Health Sciences Literature (LILACS), National Library of Medicine (PUBMED), Virtual Health Library (BVS), Scientific Electronic Library Online (SCIELO). The following descriptors were used (DECS/MESH): ANTIBIOTICS CONTROL, HOSPITAL PHARMACY, BACTERIAL RESISTANCE in English, Portuguese and Spanish. This search used papers on antibiotic control in hospital pharmacies that best suited the objective. Sixteen articles were found in the following scientific databases: Latin American and Caribbean Health Sciences Literature (LILACS), National Library of Medicine (PUBMED), Virtual Health Library (BVS), Scientific Electronic Library Online (HEAVEN). Therefore, the impact of resistant bacteria and the indiscriminate use of antibiotics in hospitals is a global problem that has been worrying the scientific community. This problem has intensified studies aimed at effectively enabling healthcare professionals, including doctors and nurses, to use hospital infection control measures correctly and effectively - such as hand washing - as well as raising awareness about the importance and need for prudent use of antibiotics as a measure to minimize the emergence of antibiotic-resistant bacteria in the hospital environment.

KEYWORDS: Pharmacy. Bacterial resistance. Antibiotics.

ABSTRACT

Brazil, in the 1980s, was initiated by the control of the first stages of health control, initiating the first process of activation of the IH Control Commissions, starting as the first the Hospital Infection Control Commissions. The main objective of the study is to evaluate the control of medicines in the hospital pharmacy. This is an integrative review, with an analytical and explanatory objective with a qualitative approach. This research through scientific publications describes its results, explaining its causes and effects. The data were published in the National Library of Health Sciences, National Scientific Health Library - (BVS Electronic Library Online (SCIELO). The following descriptors (DECS/MESH) were used: ANTIBIOTIC CONTROL, HOSPITAL PHARMACY, BACTERIAL RESISTANCE in English, Portuguese and Spanish. We used in this research the works on antibiotic control in the hospital pharmacy that best fit the objective. A total of 16 articles were found in the scientific bases: Latin American and Caribbean Literature on Health Sciences (LILACS), National Library of Medicine (PUBMED), Virtual Health Library - (BVS), Scientific Electronic Library Online (SCIELO) Therefore, the impact of resistant bacteria and the indiscriminate use of antibiotics in hospitals is a worldwide problem that worries the scientific community. This problem has intensified the search for hospital health among them, hands and health professionals, doctors and nurses. Firstly, the correct and effective use of hospital infection control measures such as washing hands - as well as making them aware of the importance and need for prudent use of antibiotics to minimize the emergence of antibiotic-resistant bacteria in the hospital environment.

KEYWORDS: Pharmacy. Bacterial resistance. Antibiotics.

SUMMARY

In the 1980s, Brazil was marked by advances in the control of HI, which began to generate awareness among health professionals, where the first Hospital Infection Control Committees emerged. The main objective of this study is to evaluate publications on antibiotic control in hospital pharmacy. The data was collected from scientific databases: Literatura Latinoamericana y del Caribe en Ciencias de la Salud (LILACS), Biblioteca Nacional de Medicina (PUBMED), Biblioteca Virtual en Salud - (BVS), Biblioteca Científica Electrónica en Línea (SCIELO). The following descriptors were used (DECS/MESH): CONTROL OF ANTIBIOTICS, HOSPITAL PHARMACY, BACTERIAL RESISTANCE in English, Portuguese and Spanish. This research used the work on antibiotic control in hospital pharmacies that best suited the objective. Sixteen articles were found in scientific databases: Literatura Latinoamericana y del Caribe en Ciencias de la Salud (LILACS), Biblioteca Nacional de Medicina (PUBMED), Biblioteca Virtual en Salud - (BVS), Biblioteca Científica Electrónica en Línea (HEAVEN). Therefore, the impact of resistant bacteria and the indiscriminate use of antibiotics in hospitals is a global problem that has been worrying the scientific community. This problem has intensified studies in the quest to effectively enable health professionals, including doctors and nurses, to use hospital infection control measures correctly and effectively - such as hand washing - as well as to raise awareness about the importance and need for prudent use of antibiotics as a measure to minimize the appearance of antibiotic-resistant bacteria in the hospital environment.

PALABRAS CLAVE: Pharmacy. Bacterial resistance. Antibiotics.

1 INTRODUCTION

In the mid-19th century, with the existence of the first hospitals, there were the first reports of HI (hospital-acquired infection), due to the high rate of epidemic diseases that attacked the poorer population. The lack of hygiene and basic sanitation was one of the main factors responsible for infection (STORPIRTIS; et al., 2008).

According to the Ministry of Health, HI is acquired after a patient enters hospital and manifests itself throughout the patient's stay or after discharge. The hospital environment often receives resistant infectious agents due to indiscriminate use, and resistance to antimicrobials affects weakened individuals who are susceptible to infection. Invasive procedures provide an environment for the spread of HI, and contaminating agents can spread to the healthcare team (GUIMARÃES; HORÁCIO; TERRA, 2017).

In the 1980s, Brazil was marked by progress in the control of HI, and the awareness of health professionals began, where the first Hospital Infection Control Commissions (CCIH) emerged (PRIMO; et al., 2010).

Even with technological scientific advances, such as the creation of new drugs and the reduction of invasive procedures, HI is still known as a serious public health problem. The high costs of treating patients and bacterial resistance to various antimicrobials make it difficult to take measures to combat infections, despite the importance of preventing and controlling these agents. Pharmaceutical activity in the hospital setting has involved a series of activities to solve the problems and difficulties encountered in the profession. The objectives of the hospital pharmacy are to ensure the rational and safe use of medicines, meet the demand for medicines, dispensing, storage and guidance for inpatients (SANTOS; GONÇALVES, 2009).

The pharmacist's duties in HI range from reducing the transmission of infections, continuous educational measures for the healthcare team and patients, to promoting the rational use of antibiotics (OLIVEIRA; PIRES, 2016).

The *marketing* of antibiotics, promoted mainly by the pharmaceutical industry, to sell these drugs as effective in fighting bacterial infections continues apace throughout the world. As a result, new broad-spectrum antibiotics have been introduced into the medical clinic. So how important is antibiotic control in the hospital environment? How important is the pharmacist in this situation?

The main objective of this study is to evaluate publications on the control of antibiotics in the hospital pharmacy. And specific objectives: to evaluate the control of the release of drugs within the hospital environment, to analyze the importance of the pharmacist in this control, to evaluate the importance of this control in reducing bacterial resistance and to analyze the importance of knowledge of these drugs.

2 METHODOLOGY

This is an integrative review, with an analytical and explanatory objective and a qualitative approach. This research seeks through scientific publications to describe its results, explaining its causes and effects (KAUARK, 2010; PEREIRA, 2018).

Data was collected using the following scientific databases: *Latin American and Caribbean Health Sciences Literature (LILACS), National Library of Medicine (PUBMED), Virtual Health Library (BVS), Scientific Electronic Library Online (SCIELO).*

The following descriptors were used (DECS/MESH)*: CONTROL OF ANTIBIOTICS, HOSPITAL PHARMACY, BACTERIAL RESISTANCE* in the following languages

English, Portuguese and Spanish. The papers on antibiotic control in the hospital pharmacy that most closely matched the objective were used in this study. All other papers and publications that were not related to the subject of this study were excluded.

The published studies were then analyzed and compared for greater relevance of the results and to evaluate the control of antibiotics in the hospital pharmacy.

The research did not present any risk, as all the data collected is provided by scientific bases.

3 RESULTS AND DISCUSSION

A total of 16 articles were found in the following scientific databases: Latin American and Caribbean Literature in Health Sciences (LILACS), *National Library of Medicine* (PUBMED), Virtual Health Library (BVS), *Scientific Electronic Library Online* (SCIELO).

3.1 Main causes of hospital-acquired infections

The hospital environment is a characteristic place for patients with different pathologies, which contributes to the spread of microorganisms present in the hospital area. Thus, the hospital ends up manifesting the risk of high-risk contamination to the hospital and especially to the patients (GUIMARÃES; HORÁCIO; TERRA, 2017).

One of the ways in which microorganisms are contaminated is through the hands of healthcare professionals towards patients, which leads to an increase in microbial growth, making these microorganisms resistant. This is due to professionals not having the habit of washing their hands properly, such as when administering medication or venipuncture, in order to aseptically clean the area and, as a consequence, control hospital infections (GUIMARÃES; HORÁCIO; TERRA, 2017).

According to Espindola (2015), the *Institute of Health Care Improvement* points to a package of infection control measures as a method of improving the processes and results of patient care, thus contributing to an improvement in the patient's clinical condition.

3.2 Common pathogens in hospital-acquired infections

The causative agents of hospital-acquired infections are bacteria, viruses, fungi and protozoa, but bacteria are the most common, such as gram-negative bacteria and those resistant to antimicrobials, while viruses and fungi are more widespread in hospital-acquired infections (SOUZA, 2014).

The main hospital infections that can be mentioned are those related to the urinary tract, respiratory tract, surgical sites and those related to the bloodstream, which in most cases are related to some invasive device, Most hospital infections are caused by bacteria, with only 20% of these infections being viral. However, infections caused by fungal agents have been on the increase over the years, and the most common infections are caused by viruses and gram-positive and gram-negative bacteria. These infectious agents include: *Staphylococcus aureus* in surgical wounds, *dermis* and blood circulation, *Staphylococcus epidermidis* in bloodstream infections, *Enterococcus* in urinary, respiratory and bloodstream infections, *Escherichia coli and Klebsiella* related to pneumonia (GUIMARÃES; HORÁCIO; TERRA, p.82, 2017).

3.3 The indiscriminate use of antibiotics

Antibiotics are drugs designed to inhibit, stop or even kill these microorganisms. However, the indiscriminate use of this medication can lead to the spread and resistance of these microorganisms (VASCONCELOS; OLIVEIRA; ARAUJO, 2015).

According to the studies carried out by Maier and Abegg (2007), the use of antibiotics should only be carried out after an antibiogram or by laboratory tests, so that the patient makes use of this medication and to treat with the correct antibiotic, since, through tests, it is possible to identify the etiological agent and consequently avoid bacterial resistance to the organism, these factors directly interfere in the quality of the patient's treatment (QUIRINO; MENDES, 2016, p. 15).

According to Quirino and Mendes (2015), when the antibiotic prescription is chosen, it is up to the pharmacist to provide guidance and pharmaceutical assistance regarding the use of this medication, which favors the patient's treatment.

3.4 Antibiotic therapy in the hospital environment and bacterial resistance

In hospitals, the uncontrolled use of antibiotics in hospitalized patients is quite common, which requires greater supervision of the use of antibiotics and consequently control over the correct administration of these drugs. This is a determining factor when it comes to bacterial resistance, as it generates problems in hospitals in general, due to bacterial resistance, which has been advancing more and more and it is important to acquire improvements in the hospital service as measures to control it (STORPIRTIS; et al., 2008).

Since antibiotics are in high demand in hospitals, one of the problems, in addition to bacterial resistance, is the cause of Adverse Drug Reactions (ADRs), which occur due to incorrect use of medication, which is common when it comes to patients who are treated with several medications (QUIRINO; MENDES, 2016).

3.5 The role of the pharmacist in the hospital pharmacy

Previously, hospital pharmacists were only recognized in pharmacies, and in the other areas where they performed their duties, they were abandoned. However, the pharmacist has been gaining ground as a professional in the distribution of medicines, as it is the pharmacist's responsibility to apply their knowledge of medicines, especially the use of antimicrobials, which requires caution in their use and administration, thus contributing to the control of the use of antimicrobials (STORPIRTIS; et al., 2008).

According to Quirino and Mendes (2016), pharmacists can provide pharmaceutical care to patients, advising them on the use of medicines, especially antibiotics, which cause bacterial resistance. According to the sole paragraph of RESOLUTION No. 585 (2013), the pharmacist's clinical attributions aim to provide care to the patient, family and community, in order to promote the rational use of medicines and optimize pharmacotherapy, with the purpose of achieving defined results that improve the patient's quality of life.

3.6 Pharmaceutical professionals in hospital infection control

According to Oliveira and Melo (2011) there is still disorientation among professionals in the hospital, problems related to prescribing medication, lack of attention when checking and problems in preparing the medication before it is administered. The choice of antimicrobial drug must be proven to be therapeutically effective for a given pathology, and it is suggested that the choice be made in conjunction with the ICHR, with the aim of controlled use of antibiotics and thus avoiding resistance from these microorganisms (BRASIL, 1994).

Initially, the choice of antibiotic is made by means of prescriptions drawn up by the doctor, with the aim of providing the best treatment for the patient. During this process, prescription errors can be avoided by working together with the team of nurses, pharmacists and the doctor to control prescription errors (OLIVEIRA; MELO, 2011).

Therefore, the participation of the pharmacist in the hospital environment allows for improvements in hospital infection control, because according to Rosa and Pinedo (2013), it is up to the pharmaceutical professional to develop their cooperation with the medicines established by the hospital such as: antimicrobials, antiseptics, cleaning and sterilizing products, together with the team of other pharmaceutical professionals.

3.7 Control of Antimicrobial Prescriptions by the CCIH (Hospital Infection Control Commission).

With the help of the pharmacist, antimicrobial prescriptions must be controlled in order to control hospital-acquired infections, because the control of prescriptions is associated with the dispensing of antimicrobials, so once these drugs are not dispensed correctly, this factor leads to problems related to microorganism resistance and worsens the patient's clinical condition (BRASIL, 1994).

In addition, there are other problematic factors regarding the use of antimicrobials, ranging from diagnostic errors mistaking bacteria for viruses to prescription errors regarding their administration, in which these barriers directly influence the quality of patient treatment and further aggravate the growth of bacteria with high resistant potential (OLIVEIRA; PIRES, 2016).

3.8 Measures adopted to control hospital-acquired infections

In the rational use of antimicrobials, the pharmacist is responsible for the correct use of these drugs, identifying the main health problems of the patient, favoring the patient's therapy (GUEDES; ALVARES, 2014).

With this, the pharmacist present in the hospital environment becomes responsible and trained to evaluate the hospital's prescriptions, provide the rational use of antimicrobials and with the help of a team of professionals, provide a pharmaceutical protocol guide, to standardize these antimicrobials that are used in the hospital, carry out tests, such as antibiograms, for the correct use of the antibiotic to treat the patient, carry out pharmaceutical care regarding the use of these drugs, prepare consumption reports and carry out training with health professionals for the prevention and elimination of microorganisms (FRANCO; MENDES; CABRAL; MENEZES, 2015).

As for the orientation of antimicrobial drug prescriptions, this is practiced by health professionals such as the prescribing doctor or the infectious disease specialist at the CCIH. However, it is up to the pharmacist to carry out this function, as he is a professional who has knowledge about medicines and purposes related to pharmaceutical care for the patient, which in fact these guidelines are not carried out by a pharmacist, because in cases of doubts about the choice of antibiotic for better therapy for the patient, the team of professionals must join the pharmacist to solve the choice of this medication, generating better quality for the patient and contributing to the proper use of antibiotics (OLIVEIRA; PIRES, 2016).

Rationalizing the use of antimicrobials is a set of actions that make it possible to improve the quality of the prescription of these drugs, based on the use of antimicrobials that offer safety for the success of the established therapy or prophylaxis, are well tolerated and cause fewer adverse effects, exerting less selective pressure on the patient's bacterial flora (GUEDES; ALVARES, 2014).

According to Oliveira and Munarreto (2010), in addition to the problems mentioned above, there are other problems, such as the unnecessary use of antibiotics and the inadequate dosage of these drugs. Another recurring factor is that during the first few hours of antibiotic use, there is the false impression that the patient no longer has the pathology, which most often leads to abandonment of treatment, favoring the growth of these microorganisms and consequently the resistance of this antibiotic (OLIVEIRA; MUNARRETO, 2010).

Due to the resistance of microorganisms, the use of antimicrobials as a choice requires a more elaborate process, as it involves pharmacological knowledge of the drug and the pathogens, as well as laboratory tests. Therefore, the choice of this drug must be made by a professional who meets these standards of excellence, which is a challenge for doctors and pharmacists. The pharmacist's role is to advise on the rational use of antimicrobials, the correct use of the medication and the identification of patients' health problems (GUEDES; ALVARES, 2014).

The habit of washing hands with soap and water eliminates unstable microorganisms and reduces inhabited microorganisms, which, depending on the case, stops the spread of disease. Currently, the term "hand washing" has been replaced by "hand hygiene" because it is a procedure with more steps, moving from simple hand washing with soap and water to an antiseptic procedure, with hand rubbing and surgical antiseptic action of the hands (MOTA; et al., 2014).

The importance of hand washing in controlling the transmission of nosocomial infection is based on the ability of hands to harbor microorganisms and transfer them from one surface to another, through direct contact, skin to skin, or indirectly, through objects (SANTOS; GONÇALVES, 2009).

Hand hygiene can be used to control infections, as it is a practice that ensures patient safety and quality (PRIMO; et al., 2010).

Therefore, as a method of preventing and controlling hospital-acquired infections, other measures should be adopted that are based on adherence and encouraging health professionals to have the habit of washing their hands correctly and frequently (MOTA; et al., 2014, p. 02).

4 CONCLUSION

Antimicrobial resistance has become the main public health problem in the world, affecting all countries, developed or not. It is an inevitable consequence of the indiscriminate use of antibiotics in humans and animals. In Europe and North America, methicillin-resistant *Staphylococcus aureus* (MRSA), non-penicillin-susceptible Streptococcus *pneumoniae* (PNSSP), vancomycin-resistant Enterococci (VRE) and extended-spectrum beta-lactamase (ESBL)-producing *Enterobacteriaceae* have emerged and spread in hospitals and communities.

For this reason, the impact of resistant bacteria and the indiscriminate use of antibiotics in hospitals is a worldwide problem that has been worrying the scientific community. This problem has intensified studies in the quest to effectively enable healthcare professionals, including doctors and nurses, to use hospital infection control measures correctly and effectively - such as hand washing - as well as making them aware of the importance and need for prudent use of antibiotics as a measure to minimize the emergence of antibiotic-resistant bacteria in the hospital environment.

Since the mid-1990s, successive implementations of anti-infective therapy have become increasingly difficult due to the spread of bacterial resistance, the emergence of new pathogens and the resultant infections in immunosuppressed patients, in whom antimicrobial drugs have become less effective·

REFERENCES

GUIMARÃES, J. N. A.; HORÁCIO, B.O.; TERRA, A. T. J. A atuação do profissional farmacêutico no controle das infecções hospitalares Revista Científica da Faculdade de Educação e Meio Ambiente, v.8, n. 1, 78-89, jan.-jun., 2017.

ESPINDOLA, M. D. A. Role of the pharmacist in hospital infection control. Postgraduate monograph presented to the Educational Training Center - CCE. Recife, 2015.

SOUZA, L. P. The challenges of preventing and controlling hospital-acquired infections at an institutional level: a discussion based on an analysis of a Brazilian healthcare institution. Monograph. Ceilândia College. Brasília, 2014.

VASCONCELOS, D. V.; OLIVEIRA, T. B.; ARAUJO, L. L. N. The use of

antimicrobials in the hospital setting and the duties of the pharmacist in the hospital infection control committee (CCIH), [S.I.: s.n.], 2015.

PORTELA, A. S.; SIMÕES, M. O. S.; FOOK, S. M. L.; NETO, A. N. M.; SILVA, P. C.

D.; Medical prescription: adequate guidelines for the use of medicines Ciência e Saúde Coletiva. State University of Paraíba. University Campus. Campina Grande PB. 2010.

PRIMO, M. G. B.; RIBEIRO, L. C. M.; FIGUEIREDO, L. F. S.; SIRICO, S. C. A.;

SOUZA, M. A. Adherence to the practice of hand hygiene by health professionals at a University Hospital. Rev. Eletr. Enf., 2010.

QUIRINO, M. G.; MENDES, R. C. Importance of the pharmacist in prevention and control with the hospital infection control program team. Rev. e-ciênc. v.4, n.2, p. 12-19, 2016.

STORPIRTS, S.; MORI, A. L. P. M.; YOCHIY, A.; RIBEIRO, E.; PORTA, V. O

Pharmacist in the Hospital Infection Control Committee In: STORPIRTS, S. Ciências Farmacêuticas: Farmácia Clínica e Atenção Farmacêutica. 1. ed. Rio de Janeiro: Guanabara Koogan, 2008.

OLIVEIRA, B. L.; PIRES, E. C. R. Atribuições do farmacêutico na comissão de controle de infecções hospitalares, [S.I.: s.n.], 2016.

OLIVEIRA, K. R.; MUNARRETO, P. RATIONAL USE OF ANTIBIOTICS: Responsibility of Prescribers, Users and Dispensers. REVISTA CONTEXTO & SAÚDE IJUÍ EDITORA UNIJUÍ v. 9 n. 18, p. 43-51, 2010.

Brazil. Ministry of Health: Basic Guide to Hospital Pharmacy, 1994.

ROSA, S. L.; PINEDO, F. J. R. THE IMPORTANCE OF THE PHARMACIST IN A HOSPITAL INFECTION CONTROL PROGRAM (PCIH), [S.I.: s.n.], 2013.

GUEDES, R. A. C; ALVARES, A. C. M. The rational use of antimicrobials as prevention of bacterial resistance, [S.I.: s.n.], 2014.

FRANCO, J. M.; MENDES R. C.; CABRAL F. R. F.; MENEZES C. D. A. The Role of Pharmacist Faced with Bacterial Resistance Caused by Irrational Use of Antimicrobials. Academic Week. Fortaleza, v.1, n.72, p.1-17, 2015. Available at: <https://semanaacademica.org.br/system/files/artigos/o_papel_do_farmaceutico_frente_a_resi stencia_bacteriana_0.pdf>. Accessed on June 18, 2019.

MOTA, E. C.; BARBOSA, D. A.; SILVEIRA, B. R. M.; RABELO, T. A.; SILVA, N. M.; SILVA, P. L. N.; RIBEIRO, J. L.; SILVA, C.S.O.; GONÇALVES, R.P.F. Hand hygiene: an evaluation of the adherence and practice of health professionals in the control of hospital infections. Rev Epidemiol Control Infect. Volume 4 - Number 1 -pg. 01-06, 2014.

SANTOS, A. A. M. The Brazilian model for hospital infection control: after twenty years of legislation, where are we and where are we going? 2006. 139 f. Dissertation (Master's) - Health Sciences: Infectology and Tropical Medicine, Faculty of Medicine, Federal University of Minas Gerais, Belo Horizonte, 2006.

CHAPTER 2

THE USE OF HOMEOPATHY IN PATIENTS WITH DEPRESSION

THE USE OF HOMEOPATHY IN PATIENTS WITH DEPRESSION

THE USE OF HOMEOPATHY IN PATIENTS WITH DEPRESSION

Michelle Diana Leal Pinheiro Matos Mac Dave Cardoso Ribeiro Matos Silva

Ricardo de Araújo

Eneas Costa Junior

Kelly Maria Rêgo da Silva Dênis Rômulo Leite Furtado

SUMMARY

Homeopathy can be used in a wide variety of treatments, such as depression, but its study should report and evaluate the levels of symptom reduction, taking the perspective of health as a complex multifactor. The main objective of this study is to demonstrate the importance of homeopathy in patients with depression. The data will be collected using the scientific databases: Latin American and Caribbean literature in health sciences - *LILACS,* national center for biotechnology information - PUBMED *virtual health library - BVS, SCIELO.* All studies reporting on the use of homeopathy in patients with depression, published between 2019 and 2023, in English and Portuguese, will be used in this study. All other works that do not fit the proposed theme and publications in other languages not mentioned above will be excluded. A total of 15 articles were found in the following scientific databases: Latin American and Caribbean Health Sciences Literature (LILACS), *National Library of Medicine* (PUBMED), Virtual Health Library (VHL), *Scientific Electronic Library Online* (SCIELO). Given this context, homeopathy as an alternative therapy in the treatment of depression may have made progress, since patients are gradually accepting this treatment, which has advantages over conventional treatment, being a very varied and vast medicinal scope, with a treatment that differs from the conventional one and that makes it possible to harm the patient minimally, in relation to conventional treatment that can provide many side effects and cause dependence on the individual.

Key words: Depression. Pharmacist. Homeopathy.

KEYWORDS: Pharmacy. Bacterial resistance. Antibiotics.

ABSTRACT

Homeopathy can be used in a wide variety of treatments, such as depression, but its study must relate and evaluate the levels of symptom reduction, tending to see health as a multifactorial complex. The main objective of the work is to demonstrate the importance of homeopathy in patients with depression. The data will be collected using the scientific databases: Literatura Latinoamericana y del Caribe en Ciencias de la Salud - LILACS, Centro Nacional de Información Biotecnológica - Biblioteca Virtual en Salud PUBMED - BVS, SCIELO. This research will use all studies related to the use of homeopathy in patients with depression, published between 2019 and 2023, in the following languages: English and Portuguese. All other work that is not included in the purpose and publication in other languages not mentioned above will be excluded. A total of 15 articles were found in the scientific databases: Literatura Latinoamericana y del Caribe en Ciencias de la Salud (LILACS), Biblioteca Nacional de Medicina (PUBMED), Biblioteca Virtual en Salud - (BVS), Biblioteca Científica Electrónica en Línea (SCIELO). In this context, homeopathy, as an alternative therapy, cannot be recommended as a treatment for depression, since patients, for some years now, have been enjoying this treatment, which has advantages over conventional treatment, being a very varied and vast medicinal field, which can offer a different treatment: conventional treatment that allows minimal harm to the patient, compared to conventional treatment that can cause many side effects and make the individual become dependent.

Key words: Depression. Pharmacist. Homeopathy.

SUMMARY

Homeopathy can be used in a wide variety of treatments, as well as depression, but its study must relate and evaluate the levels of symptom reduction, tending to see health as a multifactorial complex. The main objective of the work is to demonstrate the importance of homeopathy in patients with depression. Data will be collected using the scientific bases: Latin American and Caribbean Literature in Health Sciences - LILACS, National Center for Biotechnology Information - Virtual Health Library PUBMED - VHL, SCIELO. In this investigation, all works related to the use of homeopathy in patients with depression, published between 2019 and 2023, in the languages: English and Portuguese, will be used. All other works that are not included in the finalization and publication in other languages in the items mentioned above will be excluded. You found a total of 15 articles in the scientific databases: Literatura Latinoamericana y del Caribe en Ciencias de la Salud (LILACS), Biblioteca Nacional de Medicina (PUBMED), Biblioteca Virtual en Salud - (VHL), Biblioteca Científica Electrónica en Línea (SCIELO). In this context, homeopathy as an alternative therapy cannot help any treatment for depression, as patients, for some years now, have been taking advantage of this treatment that has sales over conventional treatment, being a very varied and vast medicinal field, which can offer a different treatment: conventional treatment that allows minimal harm to the patient, compared to conventional treatment that can provide many side effects and cause the individual to become dependent.

Keywords: Depression. Pharmaceutical. Homeopathy.

1 INTRODUCTION

In most cases, homeopathic medicines are not the first choice on the list of antidepressant drugs. Allopathic medicines are the most commonly prescribed, but they have many side effects and contraindications. Homeopathy is a natural treatment that reinforces the doctor-patient relationship, highlighting them as fundamental therapeutic tools (AGÊNCIA NACIONAL DE VIGILÂNCIA SANITÁRIA, 2011).

Depression is one of the mental disorders in which alternative and complementary therapies are used the most, homeopathy being one of them. Nowadays, individuals are learning to opt for a different treatment from the conventional one, and homeopathy in the past did not have many studies in relation to this therapy, which caused the lack of knowledge of societies and insecurity in relation to the effectiveness of the treatment, many studies show that the treatment is very efficient because it has minimal side effects, and because it is low cost (CESAR, 2019).

Homeopathy had an influence on the treatment of patients diagnosed with depression. Homeopathy is an alternative medicine that aims to cure and relieve symptoms, and through research carried out for the development of this article, it is assumed that according to reports collected, the levels of side effects from this therapy are lower than those treated with conventional drugs (LOPES, 2019).

It is an alternative treatment that requires care for the individual as a whole and not just the disease itself, that is, the mind, emotions and various organs are associated, so it is relevant that only one part of the organism should not be taken into account without taking into account the totality of the individual's organism (SOARES, 2019).

It is a disease that causes great inconvenience to the population, causing significant damage to the lives of individuals and limitations in their behavior in society. Homeopathy can be used in a wide variety of treatments for depression, but its study should report and evaluate the levels of symptom reduction, taking the perspective of health as a complex multifactor. So, what is the importance of using homeopathy in patients with depression?

The main objective of this work is to demonstrate the importance of homeopathy for patients with depression. It aims to evaluate the benefits of homeopathy, evaluate its benefits for depression; analyze the use of homeopathy and its cost.

2 DEVELOPMENT

2.1 Methodology

This is a qualitative study, with descriptive and explanatory objectives and a qualitative approach. Through scientific publications, this research seeks to describe its results, explaining their causes and effects. Its approach implies that everything carried out will be qualified and quantified in order to better demonstrate the results obtained by the research. Statistics will be used to better distribute and interpret the data (KAUARK, 2010).

All publications with data on the use of homeopathy in patients with depression, official from the *world* health organization (who) and governmental, between a certain date (2019-2023) will be used.

Data will be collected using scientific databases: Latin American and Caribbean literature in health sciences - *LILACS,* National Center for Biotechnology Information - PUBMED, *Virtual Health Library - VHL, SCIELO.* The studies will be analyzed at world, national and state level; and compared for greater relevance of the results. highlighting the importance of the use of homeopathy in patients with depression, analyzed in research.

This research will use all studies that report on the use of homeopathy in patients with depression, published between 2019 and 2023, in English and Portuguese. All other studies that do not fit the proposed theme and publications in other languages not mentioned above will be excluded.

The research will not involve any risk, as all the data will be provided by scientific bases, where there will be no contact with infected individuals and no personal data will be disclosed. The research will only be an analysis of data to demonstrate the subject.

The study will not use the Brazil Platform, because no patient data will be used, but will be carried out using scientific databases with existing information on the subject. Any procedure that could harm or alter the objectives of the work will lead to the research being terminated, such as: reporting patients' names or portraying anything more than is necessary for the research, the presence of false photos or distorting any data to fit the research or anything else that could affect it directly or indirectly.

2.2 RESULTS AND DISCUSSION

A total of 15 articles were found in the following scientific databases: Latin American and Caribbean Literature in Health Sciences (LILACS), *National Library of Medicine* (PUBMED), Virtual Health Library (BVS), *Scientific Electronic Library Online* (SCIELO).

2.1 THE EMERGENCE OF HOMEOPATHY

At the end of the 18th century and the beginning of the 19th century, a very important historical milestone was the birth of Homeopathy with Samuel Hahnemann. In general terms, it was based on the following characteristics: the diagnostic process was centered on the patient and not on the disease itself, and was based on the law of similars - Similia Similibus Curentur. Hahnemann is seen as the father of homeopathy. He graduated in medicine in 1779 and practiced his profession for a few years. During his life he gradually helped humanity and the medicine of the time by translating and publishing various works. In mid-1789, he abandoned the practice of medicine and devoted himself to translating medical works. Around 1790, translating Cullen's materia medica, he made the discovery that made him the pioneer of homeopathy (TEIXEIRA, 2017).

Cullen's medical work dealt with *Cinchona officinalis* (Quina), which had properties that strengthened the stomach, which made Hahnemann feel uneasy about the experiment, because when he fell ill with malaria, he had shown some of the characteristic symptoms of gastritis. So he began toself-administer certain doses of this plant, and began to experience signs and symptoms such as tremors and thirst. He ended up becoming his own experiment, writing down and claiming his work in the phrase: "Substances that cause a kind of fever, can cure fever". Emphasizing a new discovery in the field of medicine with the key principle "Like is kind to like". This gave rise to various experiments with other plants with a possible curative power (GOUVEIA, 2020).

Starting with quinine, he began various other experiments on himself, his family members and his collaborators. However, the experiments had to be carried out on a healthy individual, analyzing the symptoms in which the substance could be used. The substances are altered into homeopathic medicines by a specialist in the field, a homeopathic pharmacist, who uses special means and strategies for development, such as dynamization, with the aim of reducing thetoxicity of the original substance and increasing its healing power. Homeopathy is a science based on four principles: the law of similars, experimentation on healthy people, minimum and dynamized doses and the single remedy (OLIVEIRA, 2019).

The law of similars, which can also be known as the principle of similitude, is based on a substance that in a healthy individual produces certain symptoms, but in adequate and well-prepared doses, in a sick person can lead to a cure. For homeopathy, the best way to obtain knowledge of the pharmacological effects of a substance is to experiment on a healthy organism, reporting all the apparent symptoms and then administering it to a sick person. However, Hahnemann observed that the same substance administered to a man would have a different effect on an animal, since animals have a different organism to humans, causing different reactions (BRASIL, 2019).

Hahnemann carried out several experiments until he reached an intriguing result, in which he took small doses of a substance and diluted it in water or alcohol, along with this he also promoted violent agitations, and when the substance was administered to a patient he could see that the symptoms had reduced and due to the low doses there was a decrease in toxicity, but there was an increase in organic reaction, through this experiment the father of homeopathy started to make use of the technique of infinitesimal and potentiated dilutions. One of the principles of homeopathy would be the administration of one substance at a time for a better evaluation, which would be the only medicine, and not several at once (GUIMARÃES, 2019).

Thus, the combination of signs and symptoms revealed by a healthy individual when experimenting with a substance is called pathogenesis. However, the medicine that the pathogenesis best coincides with the manifestations revealed by the patient. The indication of the homeopathic medicine is based on the personal and relational characteristics of the patient. However, homeopathy still causes confusion in relation to allopathy, since allopathy (all = different; patia = disease) differs from homeopathy in that it is based on a different system that is unequal to the disease the patient is suffering from, unlike homeopathy (homeo = similar; patia = disease), which seeks a cure by means of a similar cure, i.e. the same substance that is tested on a human being and triggers symptoms in that individual, will be the same drug that cures their illness (MESQUITA, 2019).

The disadvantage of using allopathic medicines can be highlighted: most medicines have some kind of side effect, i.e. the pill administered to achieve a cure for a particular disease can cause homeopathic medicines, however, are already known for their non-toxic nature, and are intended to provide treatment at the physical, emotional and mental levels. In relation to the difficulty and controversies, it is reported that nowadays, approximately 500 million people in the world use homeopathy as a therapeutic method, which is about 7% of the world's population, establishing around 7.3 billion individuals in July 2016 (SOARES, 2019).

2.2 WHAT IS DEPRESSION?

Depression is one of the most common illnesses in the world and has been with humanity for centuries. The World Health Organization (WHO) calls it the "Evil of the Century." It is a disorder that affects the individual's emotional state and begins to manifest deep sadness, lack of energy and appetite, making it a disease with a high degree of burden. Its apparent symptoms are loss of interest and pleasure in everything, pessimism and low self-esteem, which can even lead to suicide, and is very common and can be combined (EDICASE, 2017).

Depression can be classified as mild, moderate or severe, depending on the worsening of symptoms. People with mild depression struggle to carry out simple jobs and social activities, but it doesn't cause any major impairment in their overall functioning. In the case of severe depression, the individual is totally affected and is unable to continue working, doing household chores or social activities. There are cases of depression in which the person may or may not have mania, both of which can be chronic or not, i.e. occurring over a long period of time, or relapse (DUTRA, 2019).

Recurrent depressive disorder is characterized as a disorder that develops repeated depressive episodes, during which the person has a depressed mood, loss of interest and 'pleasure and decreased energy, causing a reduction in activity in general for a period of approximately two weeks. In most cases, individuals experience symptoms of anxiety, sleep and appetite disorders and may develop feelings of guilt and low self-esteem, lack of concentration (TEIXEIRA, 2020).

Bipolar affective disorder is a type of depression that most often alternates between episodes of mania and depression, interfering with episodes of normal mood. Manic episodes can be related to an exalted or irritated mood, excessive activity, inflated self-esteem, pressure to speak, accelerated thinking and reduced need for sleep (DANTAS, 2020).

2.3 HOMEOPATHIC MEDICINES FOR THE TREATMENT OF DEPRESSION

Homeopathic treatment methods have been very effective and with fewer adverse effects when compared to the traditional treatment used for depression. According to studies, the advantages of homeopathic treatment compared to patients who underwent conventional treatment, being divided into three groups for the tests, the first were combined doses (sulpiride and homeopathic complex), the second was a single dose of the drug (sulpiride only), and the third was a dose of homeopathic complex, and through this it can be reported that the conventional treatment presented some undesirable adverse effects, and the homeopathic treatment did not find even one adverse effect (MINISTERIO DA SAÚDE, 2018).

For all medication, it is necessary to be accompanied by a trained professional, who will make a correct assessment of the emotional state, so that the patient does not opt for self-medication, which is a risk to the individual's own health. Homeopathy aims to improve the quality of life of patients by providing alternative medicines aimed at curing the disease. Depression can be understood through symptoms such as irritability, feelings of guilt, hopelessness, mood swings, social withdrawal, anger and crying for no reason, the disease can also cause the patient to be very sensitive, isolated and withdrawn (LOPES, 2019).

A homeopathic treatment must analyze the individual as a whole, both physically and mentally, and homeopathic medicines act in a non-aggressive way for the patient, stimulating the body to react naturally through its own mechanisms. In one study, 15 cases treated with homeopathy were analyzed, and 93% of positive responses were obtained, with a reduction of more than 50% in the MADRS (Montgomery and Asberg Scale) score applied in the first consultation, and then in three consecutive consultations with an interval of approximately seven weeks between each consultation, obtaining the result that in only one case there was regression, requiring referral to allopathic treatment with fluoxetine (TAMANAKA, 2019).

According to the National List of Essential Medicines (RENAME), the homeopathic medicines available in the Unified Health System (SUS) are those listed in the Brazilian Homeopathic Pharmacopoeia 3rd Edition. In order for patients to have access to these medicines through the public system, they need to seek information according to the municipality where they are listed, and the service varies according to each municipality (PUSTIGLIONE, 2019).

3 CONSIDERATIONS FINAL

Considering that depression is a prominent and very important issue, studies on homeopathic treatment are still scarce. However, it is still an acceptable alternative therapy because it is a treatment that causes minimal adverse effects to the individual.

As an alternative medicine that seeks the well-being of the patient, by analyzing the signs and symptoms presented by the individual, it is possible to indicate the dynamized substance that is most effective for the treatment.

In this context, homeopathy as an alternative therapy in the treatment of depression can make progress, since patients are gradually accepting this treatment, which has advantages over conventional treatment, being a very varied and vast medicinal scope, with a treatment that differs from the conventional one and that makes it possible to harm the patient minimally, in relation to conventional treatment that can provide many side effects and cause dependence on the individual.

REFERENCES

TEIXEIRA MZ. Scientific foundation of the homeopathic healing principle in 2017;80(1/2):40-88.

PAN AMERICAN HEALTH ORGANIZATION. World Health Organization. Allopathic and Homeopathic: what they are, what they are for and the differences; 2018. [Cited 2019 Mar 17]. Available from: https://www.opas.org.br/alopatico-e-homeopatico-o-que- sao-paraque-servem-e-diferencas/

PUSTIGLIONE M, GOLDENSTEIN E, CHENCINSKI YM. Homeopathy: a brief overview of this medical specialty. Rev. Homeopathy 2017;80(1/2):1-17. [Cited 2019 Mar 17]. Available from: https://www.cremesp.org.br/pdfs/merged.pdf

CESAR AT. Preparation of homeopathic medicines. [Online publication]; 2018 [Cited 2019 Mar 18]. Available from: http://www.bvshomeopatia.org.br/saladeleitura/texto6preparomedic amentoshomeopaticos.htm

DUTRA VC. Homeopathic pharmacotechnics. Rio de Janeiro: Redetec. 2011. [cited 2019 Mar 19]. Available from: http://respostatecnica.org.br/dossietecnico/downloadsDT/NTQzNQ== 22. Ministry of Health (Br). Depression: cause, symptoms, treatment, diagnosis and prevention. 2019. [cited 2019 Mar 31]. Available from: http://portalms.saude.gov.br/saude-de-a-z/saudemental/depressao

EDICASE. Living better-depression. 15.ed. Edic Negóciosc Edit Ltda; 2017. p.24.

LOPES AC. Diagnosis and treatment. São Paulo: Manoela; 2006. [Cited 2019 Mar 18]. Available from: https://books.google.com.br/books?id=l2RzNWwHJTMC&pg=PA41 9&dq=Lycopodium+clavatum+homeopathy&hl=enBR&sa=X&ved=0ahUKEwiIk5zLh4 3hAhVfIbkGHS5XCK0Q6AEIKT AA#v=onepage&q=Lycopodium%20clavatum%20homeopathy&f=fal se BRAZIL. Ministério da Saúde. Ordinance No. 971, of May 3, 2006. Approves the National Policy for Integrative and Complementary Practices (PNPIC) in the Unified Health System. Brasília, DF: Diario Oficial Da União. 2006. [Cited 2019 Mar 28]. Available at: http://bvsms.saude.gov.br/bvs/saudelegis/gm/2006/prt0971_03_05_ 2006.html

MINISTRY OF HEALTH. Secretariat of Science, Technology and Strategic Inputs. Department of Pharmaceutical Services and Strategic Supplies. National List of Essential Medicines: RENAME 2018 [electronic resource]. Brasília, DF: Ministry of Health. 2018. [cited 2019 Mar 28]. Available from: http://bvsms.saude.gov.br/bvs/publicacoes/medicamentos_rename. pdf.

NATIONAL HEALTH SURVEILLANCE AGENCY. Brazilian Homeopathic Pharmacopoeia. 3 ed. Brasília, DF: ANVISA. 2011. [Cited 2019 Mar 28]. Available from: http://portal.anvisa.gov.br/documents/33832/259147/3a_edicao.pdf/ cb9d5888-6b7c-447b-be3c-af51aaae7ea8

DANTAS, F.. Therapeutic results of homeopathy in suspected or confirmed covid-19 patients in Brazil: protocol for a prospective observational study. Collection of the Arthur de Almeida Rezende Filho Library, 2020.

GOUVEIA, G. D. A.. Integrative practices in primary care during the COVID-19 pandemic: Santa Catarina's experience. Revista Práticas Integrativas e Complementares: Visão Holística e Multidisciplinar, v.17, n.1, p.220-235, 2020. DOI: http://doi.org/10.37885/201001890

GUIMARÃES, N. K. N.. The use of homeopathy in the treatment of depression: a narrative review. Monograph (Bachelor's Degree in Pharmacy) - Federal University of Amazonas, Manaus, 2021.

LOPES, J.; SOUZA, W. G.; RODRIGUES, A. S.; GRETZLER, V. S.. Therapy Alternative treatment for depression: homeopathic medicines. Journal of the Faculty of Education and Environment, v.10, n.1, p.123-130, 2019.

MESQUITA, M. S. L.; MACULA, B. C. M. S.. Disinformation about homeopathy in Covid-19. Revista Fontes Documentais, v.3, n.1, p.255-262, 2020.

OLIVEIRA, C. S. R.. Depression in the elderly and homeopathic treatment. ALPHA, 2019. SOARES, J. L.; SOUZA, W. G.; SOUZA, A. R.; GRETZLER, V. S.; SANTANA JUNIOR, E. J.; CARDOSO JÚNIOR, C. D. A.; NUNES, J. S.. Alternative therapy for treating depression: homeopathic medicines. Scientific Journal of the Faculty of Education and Environment, v.10, n.1, p.123130, 2019. DOI: http://doi.org/10.31072/rcf.v10iedesp.760

TAMANAKA, P. H.. Homeopathic approach to puerperal depression: case report. ALPHA/APH, 2019.

TEIXEIRA, M. Z. Clinical research protocol to evaluate the efficacy and safety of individualized homeopathic medicine in the treatment and prevention of the COVID-19 epidemic. Revista Câmara Brasileira do Livro, v.1, n.1, p.1-63, 2020.

CHAPTER 3

DRUG INTERACTIONS IN AESTHETICS: A SYSTEMATIC REVIEW

DRUG INTERACTIONS IN AESTHETICS: A SYSTEMATIC REVIEW

DRUG INTERACTIONS IN AESTHETICS: A SYSTEMATIC REVIEW

Michelle Diana Leal Pinheiro Matos Mac Dave Cardoso Ribeiro Matos Silva

Ricardo de Araújo

Eneas Costa Junior

Kelly Maria Rêgo da Silva Dênis Rômulo Leite Furtado

SUMMARY

The connection between the pharmacist and the patient undergoing considerable psychological changes is of fundamental importance in pharmaceutical care, since the pharmacist is one of those responsible for guiding rational pharmacotherapy and achieving the intended therapeutic goal. The main objective of this study is to evaluate scientific publications on the subject of drug interactions in aesthetics from 2010 to 2022. It is an integrative review, with an analytical and explanatory objective and a qualitative approach. This research seeks to describe the results of scientific publications, explaining their causes and effects. The data was collected using the following scientific databases: *Latin American and Caribbean Health Sciences Literature (LILACS), National Library of Medicine (PUBMED), Virtual Health Library (Biblioteca Virtual em Saúde).*
- (BVS), Scientific Electronic Library Online (SCIELO). The following descriptors were used (DECS/MESH): *DRUG INTERACTIONS IN AESTHETICS, PHARMACISTS IN AESTHETICS, AESTHETICS AND SIDE EFFECTS* in English, Portuguese and Spanish. This research used the papers on drug interactions in aesthetics that most closely matched the objective, published between 2010 and 2022. A total of 38 articles were found in the following scientific databases: Latin American and Caribbean Health Sciences Literature (LILACS), *National Library of Medicine* (PUBMED), Virtual Health Library (VHL), *Scientific Electronic Library Online* (SCIELO). Pharmaceutical care will therefore promote personalized, humanized and scientifically correct care.

Key words: Pharmacy. Aesthetics. Patient safety. Side effects. Drugs.

KEYWORDS: Pharmacy. Bacterial resistance. Antibiotics.

ABSTRACT

The connection between the pharmacist and the patient who undergoes a considerable psychological change is of fundamental importance in pharmaceutical care, as the pharmacist is one of those responsible for guiding rational pharmacotherapy and achieving the expected therapeutic objective. The main objective of this study is to evaluate scientific publications that address the topic of drug interactions in aesthetics from 2010 to 2022. It is an integrated review, with analytical and explanatory objectives with a qualitative approach. This investigation seeks, through scientific publications, to describe its results, explaining its causes and effects. The data was collected using scientific bases: Literatura Latinoamericana y del Caribe en Ciencias de la Salud (LILACS), Biblioteca Nacional de Medicina (PUBMED), Biblioteca Virtual en Salud - (VHL), Biblioteca Científica Electrónica en Línea (SCIELO). It can be used as descriptors (DECS/MESH): INTERACCIONES MEDICAMENTOSAS EN ESTÉTICA, FARMACÉUTICO EN ESTÉTICA, ESTÉTICA Y EFECTOS SECONDARIOS in English, Portuguese and Spanish. In this investigation, you used the works on drug interactions in aesthetics that best fit the objective, published between 2010 and 2022. You found a total of 38 articles in the scientific databases: Latin American and Caribbean Literature in Health Sciences (LILACS) , National Library of Medicine (PUBMED), Virtual Health Library - (VHL), Online Electronic Scientific Library (SCIELO). Pharmaceutical care will therefore promote personalized, humanized and scientifically correct care.

Keywords: Pharmacy. Aesthetics. Patient safety. Side effects. Drugs.

SUMMARY

The connection between the pharmacist and the patient undergoing a considerable psychological change is of fundamental importance in pharmaceutical care, since the pharmacist is one of those responsible for guiding rational pharmacotherapy and achieving the expected therapeutic objective. The main objective of this study is to evaluate scientific publications that address the issue of drug interactions in aesthetics from 2010 to 2022. It is an integrative review, with analytical and explanatory objectives and a qualitative approach. This research seeks, through scientific publications, to describe their results, explaining their causes and effects. The data was collected using scientific databases: Literatura Latinoamericana y del Caribe en Ciencias de la Salud (LILACS), Biblioteca Nacional de Medicina (PUBMED), Biblioteca Virtual en Salud - (BVS), Biblioteca Científica Electrónica en Línea (SCIELO). The following descriptors were used (DECS/MESH): MEDICINE INTERACTIONS IN ESTHETICS, PHARMACEUTICALS IN ESTHETICS,
ESTHETICS AND SECONDARY EFFECTS in English, Portuguese and Spanish. This research used the papers on drug interactions in aesthetics that best fit the objective, published between 2010 and 2022. A total of 38 articles were found in the scientific databases: Literatura Latinoamericana y del Caribe en Ciencias de la Salud (LILACS), Biblioteca Nacional de Medicina (PUBMED), Biblioteca Virtual en Salud - (BVS), Biblioteca Científica Electrónica en Línea (SCIELO). Pharmaceutical care will therefore promote personalized, humanized and scientifically correct care.

Key words: Pharmacy. Aesthetics. Patient safety. Side effects. Drugs.

1 INTRODUCTION

Pharmaceutical care" is a pharmaceutical practice developed in the context of pharmaceutical assistance. It encompasses attitudes, ethical values and commitments to disease prevention, health promotion and recovery in an integrated manner with the healthcare team. The pharmacist's direct interaction with the patient, aimed at rational pharmacotherapy and obtaining defined and measurable results aimed at improving quality of life. Appropriate pharmacotherapy and the patient's clinical and psychological condition are essential elements for the development of this pharmaceutical practice, and the use of medicines is influenced by cultural, social, economic and political factors (ALMA; COSTA, 2011).

In 1996 in Brazil, medicines ranked first among the three main agents causing poisoning in human beings. In 2008, 40% of poisoning cases in the state of São Paulo were caused by medicines and 50% of re-hospitalizations in the state of Rio de Janeiro were due to incorrect use of prescribed medicines or abandonment of treatment (SEGRE; FERRAZ, 1997).

Research carried out in different countries in North America and Europe shows a favorable impact of pharmaceutical care on effectiveness, quality of life and healthcare costs, proving to be an excellent model for the economy, especially for developing countries that have a health system with scarce financial resources (STREHLAU; CLARO; NETO, 2014).

As well as scientific training, pharmacists must have the ability to communicate with their staff and patients. In many cases, failure to follow prescriptions reflects a lack of education based on the pharmacist/patient relationship. It is therefore very important to know the level of education of patients, in order to better direct communication techniques, both oral and written, at the time of counseling (CAMARGO et al., 2011).

In the dermatological field, especially in relation to acne, the pharmacist's work must include these two factors, since, in the long term, psychological changes may develop due to the appearance of unsightly lesions or scars, leading the patient to experience considerable social discomfort, as well as anxiety and depression caused by acne, characteristics that can compromise treatment and cause social changes in the patient's life (CASTRO, 2011).

Therefore, understanding the severity of the disease is very important for guiding treatment. Acne is a chronic inflammatory condition of the sebaceous hair follicle that mainly affects the face and upper trunk. The mechanism ofacne formation involves follicular hyperkeratinization, and with it, a horny plug with sebaceous content forms inside the gland, known as a comedone or blackhead (ALMA; COSTA, 2011).

The occluded follicle facilitates the action of Propionibacterium acnes (P. acnes) and yeasts such as Pityrosporum orbiculare (P. orbiculare), which release hydrolytic proteases that rupture the cell lumen, expelling the sebum content into the dermis. Sebaceous lipids, hair, P. acnes and cornified epitheliocytes generate a foreign body-type immune response. It is classified as non-inflammatory and inflammatory, and subdivided into degrees. Non-inflammatory acne: comedonic (grade I), inflammatory acne: papulopustular (grade II), nodulocystic (grade III), conglobate (grade IV), fulminant (grade V). (CASTRO, 2011).

The connection between the pharmacist and the patient, who is undergoing considerable psychological change, is of fundamental importance in pharmaceutical care, since the pharmacist is one of those responsible for guiding rational pharmacotherapy and achieving the planned therapeutic goal. In this sense, pharmaceutical care, a patient-centered model, has emerged as an alternative in the quest to improve the quality of the process of using medicines in order to achieve concrete and satisfactory results. So, what drug interactions are present in aesthetics? And the importance of the pharmacist in this area?

The main objective of this study is to evaluate scientific publications on the subject of drug interactions in aesthetics from 2010 to 2022. It also aims to evaluate the most common drug interactions in aesthetics, assess the importance of the pharmacist in these applications, analyze the possible interactions that have occurred, analyze the best methodology to avoid drug implications and analyze the importance of knowledge of drugs for aesthetics.

2 DEVELOPMENT

2.1 Methodology

This is an integrative review, with an analytical and explanatory objective and a qualitative approach. This research seeks through scientific publications to describe its results, explaining its causes and effects (KAUARK, 2010; PEREIRA, 2018).

Data was collected using the following scientific databases: *Latin American and Caribbean Health Sciences Literature (LILACS), National Library of Medicine (PUBMED), Virtual Health Library (BVS), Scientific Electronic Library Online (SCIELO).*

The following descriptors were used (DECS/MESH): *DRUG INTERACTIONS IN AESTHETICS, PHARMACISTS IN AESTHETICS, AESTHETICS AND*

SIDE EFFECTS in English, Portuguese and Spanish. This research used the papers on drug interactions in aesthetics that best fit the objective, published between 2010 and 2022. All other studies and publications not related to the subject of this study were excluded.

The published studies were then analyzed and compared for greater relevance of the results and to evaluate drug interactions in aesthetics. The research presented no risk, as all the data collected was provided by scientific databases.

2.2 Results and Discussion

A total of 38 articles were found in the following scientific databases: Latin American and Caribbean Literature in Health Sciences (LILACS), *National Library of Medicine* (PUBMED), Virtual Health Library (BVS), *Scientific Electronic Library Online* (SCIELO).

2.2.1 Aesthetic pharmacy legislation

According to Vieira et al. (2019), aesthetic health focuses on the promotion, protection, maintenance and recovery of individual health. In this scenario, the regulation of pharmacists' work in aesthetic health has opened up a new possibility for pharmacists to promote care, as well as expanding their scope of action. The resolutions of the Federal Pharmacy Council (CFF) No. 573 of 2013, No. 616 of 2015 and No. 645 of 2017 regulate the pharmacist's work in aesthetic health. To work in this area, pharmacists must be qualified by the CRF in their jurisdiction byproving the requirements set out in Article 2 of CFF Resolution No. 616 of 2015, as amended by CFF Resolution No. 645 of 2017. Federal Pharmacy Council (CFF) Resolution No. 573 of May 22, 2013, recognizes health and aesthetics as an area in which pharmacists can work, as well as being the establishment's technical manager, as long as the established procedures do not use surgical procedure criteria. It establishes technical rules and criteria for the professional duly qualified for these activities (BRASIL, 2013).

In Resolution No. 616 of November 25, 2015, the CFF describes new aesthetic procedures that are open to professional pharmacists. However, in order to become an aesthetic pharmacist, they must be graduates of a postgraduate program in the field of aesthetic health, be graduates of a course recognized by the CFF and have at least two years' continuous experience in the field (BRASIL, 2015).

CFF Resolution No. 645 of July 27, 2017, includes two procedures that pharmacists can perform, which are self-supporting thread lifting and ablative laser therapy, and they can also have autonomy over the use and purchase of substances and equipment needed for co-aesthetic procedures (BRASIL, 2017).

2.2.2 Professional aesthetic pharmacist

The role of the professional pharmacist in aesthetic procedures is increasingly extensive, as various factors such as stretch marks, acne, localized fat, cellulite, aging marks, wrinkles and expression lines are some of the adversities that bother Brazilians who care about their appearance, thus increasing the search for aesthetic therapeutic resources. It is therefore essential to know how to assess the specific needs of each patient, providing a differentiated service, obtaining recognition and appreciation for your professional (FERNANDES; NASCIMENTO; GUALBERTO, 2019).

The success of the pharmacist in the field of aesthetics is linked to the knowledge obtained during their undergraduate studies, enabling them to carry out patient anamnesis, identifying skin biotypes and aesthetic dysfunctions, providing pharmaceutical care services and indicating non-prescription drugs for the treatment of skin pathologies, improving the patient's quality of life (SILVA; MERCADO, 2015).

The growth of the cosmetology and esthetics market is notorious, so there is a need for professionals to update and deepen their knowledge, expanding their capacity and skills to guarantee quality services. In this way, pharmacists are able to work in aesthetic establishments and clinics, playing an essential role in the basic care of chronic and non-communicable diseases, providing guidance on the rational use of medicines, identifying possible interactions between drug therapy and aesthetic treatment (CRIPPA, 2016).

In view of the above, the aesthetic pharmacist offers effective treatment and patient safety, as he is a health professional who is trained, specialized and qualified for such aesthetic procedures, always putting the patient's health first. They also advise on the correct use of medication, allowing the appropriate choice of products in relation to the aesthetic therapy recommended to the patient, thus leading to better adherence to their therapy (ALMA; COSTA, 2011).

2.2.3 Pharmaceutical care for health and aesthetics

Pharmaceutical care is an exclusive competence of the pharmaceutical professional. It is based mainly on the patient's pharmacotherapeutic care, seeking satisfactory results through problem solving and guidance on the rational use of medicines, avoiding possible Drug-Related Problems (DRPs) (CARDOSO et al., 2013).

When pharmaceutical professionals combine the practices of pharmaceutical health care and aesthetics, they achieve excellent results, as they provide counseling and follow-up, adapting the best aesthetic therapy for each patient, as well as closely monitoring drug therapy, obtaining satisfactory treatment results (PEREIRA; FREITAS, 2008). Therefore, pharmacists should continuously seek improvements in their technical work circumstances, to provide a safe environment for the patient, and pharmaceutical care is extremely important to achieve success in aesthetic therapy, highlighting the quality of life of patients by directly intervening in their self-esteem and well-being (OLIVEIRA, 2017).

2.2.4 The pharmacist's role in aesthetics with an emphasis on ageing

Aesthetic pharmacists promote individual health and provide aesthetic corrections, using resources that improve the quality of life of their users, but these procedures must not be invasive and must follow the standards required by the CFF (BRASIL, 2018).

It is important to emphasize the importance of such professionals in this highly competitive area. Pharmacists stand out in this market because they have extensive physiological knowledge and the ability to create their own cosmetics, thus providing a differentiated and personalized service, prescribing and producing more effective products (GODOY et al., 2016).

Among the many duties of the pharmacist in aesthetics, some are highlighted because they are on the rise in the world of influencers, such as chemical and mechanical peeling, sonophoresis (aesthetics, ionophoresis, cryolipolysis, aesthetic ultrasound), radiofrequency carboxytherapy, botulinum toxin, intradermal therapy/mesotherapy, ablative laser therapy, as well as aesthetic assessment and counseling (VENDRAMINI, 2018).

The population sees aging as something to be combated, they want to maintain a more youthful appearance, and so they seek out anti-aging treatments. Among the most sought-after procedures is the application of botulinum toxin, which is capable of causing muscle paralysis, softening the appearance of expression lines and wrinkles, followed by treatment with chemical peeling, which is a process that causes lesions in the skin, thus stimulating cell regeneration with the help of some acids, such as glycolic acid, retinoic acid, among others, and finally the use of topical cosmetics containing antioxidant substances in their formulation (SCOTTI et al., 2007).

2.2.5 Botulinum toxin

The aesthetics market is mainly driven by what is fashionable, but there are aesthetic practices that will never cease to exist. Expression lines have always been the dreaded villains and are responsible for the demand for one of the five most popular aesthetic procedures on the market, the so-called botulinum toxin (CIDREIRA, 20 08). Popularly known as botox, *botulinum* toxin is produced by a microorganism called *Clostridium botulinum*. It is a bacterium that needs to be isolated and purified in order to be used. This bacterium is responsible for reducing muscle hypertonia and inhibiting the release of acetylcholine at the nerve endings. pre used on the market is type A (bontsynaptic. Botulinum toxin plus A), which is mainly applied to reduce wrinkles and facial expression lines. However, this toxin is not only used for aesthetic purposes, but also to treat some symptoms of degenerative diseases (NOGUEIRA, 2016).

According to Resolution No. 616 of 2015, pharmacists are able to perform the minimally invasive botulinum toxin application procedure, since this practice is a non-surgical injection, so pharmacists can perform this procedure (BRASIL, 2015).

Since then, pharmaceutical professionals have increasingly sought specialization in the field of aesthetics, many of them with the aim of perfecting their botulinum toxin techniques. The demand for this type of procedure is due to its low risk, making it highly accepted by aesthetic procedure enthusiasts. With pharmaceutical monitoring, these risks are even lower, as adverse reactions can be avoided, resulting in even better results for the user (LIMA, 2017).

Some pharmacological attributions allow us to say that pharmacists have advantages in the application of botulinum toxin over other professionals who are also qualified to perform these procedures, such as the correct form of storage and conservation, preparation and dilution of the dose to be applied, quantity of the correct dose, as well as knowing exactly what the contraindications are, supra dosage and interactions that botulinum toxin has in relation to other medication (MENEGASSO et al., 2016).

Pharmacists, in their many roles, insistently seek to avoid DRPs (Drug-Related Problems), most of which occur due todrug interactions, which can be avoided with care, guidance and pharmaceutical interventions (ZANELLA; ASSINI, 2008).

Botulinum toxin is no different; its effect can be altered depending on the interaction with other drugs. We can mention the potentiation of the toxin when associated with drugs that act on the neuro junction, which can be antibiotics and muscle calcium blockers. Individuals who use these drugs need to be more closely observed and receive extra care when treated with botulinum toxin (SPOSITO, 2014).

In addition, botulinum toxin is not only sought after for facial fillers, it can also be used in other procedures such as strabismus, blepharospasm, spasticity, hyperhidrosis, cerebral palsy, hemifacial spasm, cervical and limb dystonia, bruxism, gummy smile, tremors, persistent contraction of the chewing muscles, myofacial pain syndrome, neuromuscular dysfunctions, among others (RIBEIRO et al., 2014).

2.2.6 Chemical Peeling

Peels are aesthetic procedures carried out with the aim of refining the skin and promoting cell renewal, limiting superficial wrinkles. The aesthetic pharmacist is the professional who can carry out this type of procedure, including chemical, mechanical and physical peels (TESTON; NARDINO, 2010).

Chemo exfoliation is based on the application of exfoliating agents to the skin, such as acids, resulting in the degradation of cells in the dermis or epidermis, followed by cell regeneration, normalizing pigmentation and reducing wrinkles and blemishes. This treatment is commonly used for skin therapy caused by sun damage, facial wrinkles, melasma, pigmentary dyschromias, acne scars, hyperpigmentation, and hair with enlarged pores (WEICK, 2002).

Thus, chemical peels are classified into three types of procedure: superficial, medium and deep. Superficial peels act on the epidermis and are indicated for the treatment of acne, hyperkeratotic aczema, photoaging, actinic keratosis, melasma and fine wrinkles. Medium peels act on the papillary dermis and have the same uses as superficial peels, but are indicated for epidermal lesions. Finally, the deep peel acts on the reticular dermis and is indicated for blemishes, epidermal lesions, actinic dyschromias, scars, keratosis, moderate wrinkles, lentigos and melasma (VELASCO et al., 2004).

The demand for this method has been growing, given its effectiveness in the treatment outcome, and the professional pharmacist stands out for being a trained professional to perform this procedure, in view of his knowledge in the pharmacological area so that there are no adverse reactions in the treatment such as adverse reactions to chemical agents, allergic reaction and toxicity (BORGES; SILVA, 2019).

It's important to note that care after chemical peeling procedures should be guided by pharmaceutical professionals, such as avoiding exposure to sunlight, applying sunscreens daily, moisturizing several times a day and using neutral soaps suitable for the face. These methods contribute to the final effectiveness of the treatment using chemical peels (RAMOS, 2004).

2.2.7 Cosmetotherapy

When we use topical applications of substances that have therapeutic and aesthetic purposes in their formulation, we are talking about cosmetotherapy. It is important to pay attention to the concentration and quantity of products to be applied to each individual, so it is extremely important that the professional has skills and mastery of the drug used, its usual construction and the specific conditions of each user (MORAES et al., 2017).

The worldwide concern of individuals with premature aging has led to a considerable increase in the use of cosmetics in recent years, resulting in major investments by industries in the manufacture of a wide range of products for cosmetic therapeutic purposes. In this context, there are various dermatological products used to treat acne, dehydration, ageing, blemishes, cellulite, stretch marks, among others (PAULA, 2013).

Pharmacists have a great advantage in this area, given that the products used for cosmetotherapy are generally studied, manufactured and supervised by pharmaceutical professionals, who in their academic training acquire specific knowledge for the formulation of drugs and cosmetics in general.

In view of this, the pharmaceutical professional has knowledge of the appropriate cosmeceuticals for use in each specific treatment, knowing how to conduct the best aesthetic treatment, leading to better results (HASHIMOTO; BARROS, 2018).

2.2.8 Aesthetic Health Pharmaceutical Establishment

Resolution 573 of 2013 brought a great achievement for the professional pharmacist, as this resolution allowed not only the professional to carry out aesthetic activities, but also the release of technical responsibility for aesthetic establishments by pharmacists (BRASIL, 2013).

Just like any other establishment that provides health care to the population, the opening of an aesthetic clinic under pharmaceutical responsibility is no different. The pharmacist acting as the technical manager of the establishment in question must meet all the requirements imposed by Law 9.078/90, which are established in order to provide the best service to the individual (TELES, 2012).

Law 8078 of 1990 defines the rules that protect the consumer in the face of a service provision, aiming to protect the rights of the consumer, as well as clarifying the relationships and responsibilities between the service provider and the consumer, leading to guarantees of a quality service. (BRASIL, 1990).

In addition, it is mandatory that when pharmacists have technical responsibility for an aesthetic establishment, they strictly follow the determinations imposed by Resolution 573 of May 22, 2013, and the other resolutions following it, thus ensuring credibility and appreciation for the establishment, providing better results for users of aesthetic services (BRASIL, 2013).

2.2.9 Drug interactions

Acne is mainly treated using antimicrobials, retinoids and abrasive agents. Antimicrobials are compounds that in low concentrations inhibit or reduce the growth of various microorganisms. Among these, the most commonly used in acne treatment are azelaic acid and benzoyl peroxide (STREHLAU; CLARO; NETO, 2014).

In topical preparations, azelaic acid has a hypopigmenting effect and can cause local irritation and photosensitization as an adverse effect. It is not considered a first-choice treatment, but it is a good alternative for mild to moderate acne or acne with post-inflammatory hyperpigmentation (ALMA; COSTA, 2011).

It is relatively non-toxic and there is no evidence of drug interaction with other drugs due to its low systemic absorption. As for how to use it, two applications a day are recommended on the affected skin in the form of a cream or gel between

5 % to 15 % for six months. Its use with benzoyl peroxide, clindamycin, tretinoin or erythromycin increases its effectiveness (ZANELLA; ASSINI, 2008).

Benzoyl peroxide has a drying and peeling activity, which helps its efficacy. It should not be applied to irritated skin or to skin burnt by wind or sun. It is not recommended for people who are hypersensitive to this substance. The most common adverse effects are dryness, hardening of the skin and a burning sensation. It is not recommended to be applied together with topical preparations such as retinoids and antibiotics due to their irritating effect (CAMARGO et al., 2011).

It is commercially available in gel and cream form in concentrations of1

It can be used on the affected skin once or twice a day. Antimicrobial agents also include antibiotics, which are used for bacterial infections. Antibiotics are usually prescribed in cases of moderate to severe acne. These include tetracycline, used systemically, erythromycin both topically and systemically and clindamycin only topically (CASTRO, 2011).

The main adverse effects of these drugs are gastrointestinal disorders, as well as induction of resistance, so their use schedule must be strictly adhered to. Tetracycline was, for a long time, the drug of choice for acne therapy, due to its efficacy, tolerance and high safety margin. However, it is no longer prevalent due to its adverse effects and interactions with other drugs (FERNANDES; NASCIMENTO; GUALBERTO, 2019).

The adverse effects attributed to the use of tetracycline are kidney disorders, photosensitivity, increased levels of liver enzymes producing hepatotoxicity, pancreatitis, central nervous system toxicity, pseudomembranous colitis, hypersensitivity reactions and Candida vaginitis. Antacids, milk and foods containing calcium, magnesium and iron should also not be used during treatment, as they form complexes with tetracycline, reducing its absorption (CRIPPA, 2016).

Combination with retinoids can cause intracranial hypertension. Nephrotoxic effects are enhanced in combination with methoxyflurane and other diuretics that have nephrotoxicity as an adverse effect. Generally, doses of 500 mg of tetracycline twice a day are indicated. Tetracycline is contraindicated in liver and kidney failure, pregnancy and children. The use of tetracycline between the 2nd trimester of pregnancy and around 8 years of age is also contraindicated, due to the fixation of the drug on developing teeth, causing color changes and hypoplasia (VELASCO et al., 2004).

3 CONSIDERATIONS FINAL

Vanity is directly associated with an individual's health and aesthetics, as it has a direct impact on their self-esteem and well-being, leading to greater consumption of cosmetics and aesthetic treatments, with the aim of improving their body and beauty, resulting in mental and physical self-fulfillment.

Recent research on the body has shown that aesthetics is gradually becoming a problem, caused by the inducement of the media, such as magazines and television, to produce standards of beauty and health, creating feelings of anguish and shock in individuals, encouraging them to seek the perfect body aesthetic and maintain their health.

The pharmacist who works in this area must keep up with the development of beauty worldwide, promoting aesthetic solutions and appropriate facial and body therapeutic resources, not forgetting health as a primary benefit, since society targets beauty standards as survival factors.

As there is a wide variety of drugs used to treat acne, some with potential toxicity, the relationship between pharmacist and patient is essential for successful pharmacotherapy. Clear information on the best way to carry out treatment, using medicines correctly and clarifying possible adverse reactions and drug interactions, will effectively help to minimize the risks of self-medication, drug poisoning and treatment abandonment. Pharmaceutical care will therefore promote personalized, humanized and scientifically correct care.

REFERENCES

ALMA, Jeanete Moussa; COSTA, Magda Lucy Ribeiro Botelho da. The media world in

the world of beauty: how beauticians acquire their cosmetic products.
Revista Brasileira de Ciências Farmacêuticas, v. 10, n. 5, p. 166187, 2011. ALVES, HérickHebert da Silva et al. The pharmacist's role in aesthetic health. **Scientific Exhibition of Pharmacy**, 2016.

BARROS, Mateus Domingues de; OLIVEIRA, Rita Patrícia Almeida de. Aesthetic treatment and the concept of beauty. **Biological and Health Sciences**, v. 3, n. 1, p. 65-74, 2017.

BORGES, Isabela Sousa; SILVA, Cláudia Peres da. Chemical peeling in the treatment of photoaged hands. **Humanidades & Tecnologia em Revista**, v. 16, p.
1809-1628, 2019.

BORBA, Tamila; THIVES, Fabiana Marin. A reflection on the influence of aesthetics on human self-esteem, self-motivation and well-being. **Revista de Farmácia**, Santa Catarina. p. 1-21, 2018.

BRAZIL. Ministry of Health, Law No. 8.078, of September 11, 1990. Brasília. BRASIL. Ministério da Saúde, RDC n 573, of May 22, 2013. Brasília. BRAZIL. Ministry of Health, RDC no. 645, of July 27, 2017. Brasília.

BRAZIL. Ministry of Health, RDC No. 669, of December 13, 2018. Brasília.

CAMARGO, Brigido Vizeu et al. Social representations of the body: aesthetics and health. **Temas em Psicologia**, Santa Catarina, v. 19, n. 1, p. 257 - 268, 2011.

CASTRO, Ana Lucia de. Health and aesthetics: the medicalization of beauty. **Revista Eletrônica de Comunicação Inovação e Saúde**, Rio de Janeiro, v. 5, n. 4, p. 14-23, 2011.

CIDREIRA, Renata Pitombo. Fashion and style: an introduction to the aesthetics of fashion.
Revista FAMECOS, Porto Alegre, n. 36, p. 48-53, 2008.

CLAUDIA, Serafin; JÚNIOR, Daniel Correia; VARGAS, Mirella. Profile of pharmacists in Brazil: report. Federal Pharmacy Council, Brasília, 44.p, 2015. CRIPPA, Valdinara de Oliveira. Non-invasive techniques for reducing localized lipodystrophy: current evidence. Emphasis on treatment with cryolipolysis. **Infarma Ciências Farmacêuticas**, v. 28, n. 4, p. 1999-2007, 2016.

FERNANDES, Diego da Silva; NASCIMENTO, Derina Martins; GUALBERTO, Amanda C. Assis. Technological innovations and the role of pharmacists in the anti-aging

process. **Revista Educação Meio Ambiente e Saúde**, Rio de Janeiro, v. 9, n. 1, 2019.
GODOY, Isabela Martins et al. The pharmacist's role in aesthetic health. **Revista Eletrônica de Trabalhos Acadêmicos**, Goiânia, p. 1-15, 2016.
HASHIMOTO, Hevelly Hydeko; BARROS, Kleber Vânio Gomes. Quality Assurance in the Production Area of a Cosmetics Industry. Pontifical Catholic University of Goiás, Goiás, p. 18, 2018.

LIMA, Juliana Rodrigues. Therapeutic resources used by pharmacists in aesthetic health. **Saúde Coletiva**, Ariquemes, 2017.
MENEGASSO, Pedro Eduardo et al. Aesthetic pharmacy. Regional Pharmacy Council of São Paulo, p. 129-145, 2016.
MORAES, Amanda Luzia Soares de et al. Cosmetology: origin, evolution and trends. **Brazilian Cosmetics Magazine,** 2017.
NOGUEIRA, Carlla Luanna de Carvalho. The application of botulinum toxin type a in the
treatment of the signs of facial skin aging. **Saúde Coletiva**, Recife, 2016. PAULA, Carolina Costa de. Pre-formulation studies and development of cosmetics - FloraBrasil line. **Ciência & Saúde Coletiva**, Araraquara, p. 44, 2013.
PEREIRA, Leonardo Régis Leira; FREITAS, Osvaldo de. The evolution of pharmaceutical care and the outlook for Brazil. **Revista Brasileira de Ciências Farmacêuticas**, São Paulo, v. 44, n. 4, p. 602-612, 2008.
PEREIRA, Mariana Linhares; NASCIMENTO, Mariana Martins Gonzaga do. From apothecaries to pharmaceutical care: perspectives of the pharmaceutical professional. **Revista Brasileira de Farmácia**, Minas Gerais, p. 245-252, 2011.
RAMOS, Tatiane Rodrigues. Validation of analytical methodologies for the quantitative determination of active ingredients in pharmaceutical formulations for chemical peels. **Ciência & Saúde Coletiva**, São Paulo, 2004.
RIBEIRO, Isar Naves De Souza et al. The use of botulinum toxin type "a" in dynamic wrinkles of the upper third of the face. **Revista da Universidade** Ibirapuera, São Paulo, v. 7, p. 31-37, 2014.
SATURNINO, Luciana Tarbes Mattana et al. Pharmacist: a professional in search of his identity. **Revista Brasileira de Farmácia,** Minas Gerais, p. 1016, 2012.
SEGRE, Marco; FERRAZ, Flávio Carvalho. The concept of health. **Revista de Saúde**

Pública, São Paulo, v. 31, n. 5, p. 538-542, 1997.

SCOTTI, Luciana et al. Molecular modeling applied to the development of molecules with antioxidant activity for cosmetic use. **Revista Brasileira de Ciências Farmacêuticas**, São Paulo, v. 43, n. 2, p. 153-166, 2007.

SILVA, Tatiane Rosa Bega da; MERCADO, Naiara Fernanda. Cryolipolysis and its efficacy in the treatment of localized fat: a literature review. **Visão Universitária**, v. 3, p. 129-145, 2015.

SPOSITO, Maria Matilde de Mello. Botulinum toxin type A - pharmacological properties and clinical use. **ActaFisiátr**, São Paulo, 2014.

STREHLAU, Vivian Iara; CLARO, Danny Pimentel; NETO, Silvio Abrahão Laban. Does vanity drive the consumption of cosmetics and aesthetic surgical procedures in women? An exploratory investigation. **Revista Adm**, São Paulo, v. 50, n. 1, p. 73-88, 2015.

TELES, Felipe Barbosa. Consumer Protection and Defense Code and Related Legislation. **Brazilian Journal of Pharmaceutical Sciences**, Brasília, n. 5, p. 109, 2012. TESTON, Ana Paula; NARDINO, Deise. Skin ageing: free radical theory and treatments for prevention and rejuvenation. Ciência & Saúde Coletiva, 2010.

VELASCO, Maria Valéria Robles et al. Skin rejuvenation by chemical peeling: focus on phenol peeling. **An bras Dermatol**, Rio de Janeiro, v. 79, n. 1, p. 91-99, 2004.

VENDRAMINI, Rochelle. Therapies used in aesthetic pharmacy professional procedures. **Brazilian Journal of Pharmaceutical Sciences**, 2018.

VIEIRA, Amanda Carla Quintas de Medeiros et al. Growth factors: a new cosmeceutical approach for anti-aging care. **Revista Brasileira de Farmácia**, v. 92, n. 3, p. 80-89, 2011.

VIEIRA, Thaiany Cavalcante et al. Pharmaceutical performance in the field of aesthetics. **Scientific Exhibition of Pharmacy**, 2019.

WEICK, Karl. The aesthetics of imperfection in orchestras and organizations. **Revista de Administração de Empresas**, São Paulo, v. 42, n. 3, p. 6-18, 2012.

ZANELLA, Vanessa; ASSINI, Fabrício Luiz. Identification of drug-related problems in geriatric patients in the city of Concórdia. **Revista Brasileira de Farmácia**, Santa Catarina, v. 89, n. 4, p. 294-297, 2008.

CHAPTER 4

THE IMPACT OF SELF-MEDICATION ON SOCIETY

THE IMPACT OF SELF-MEDICATION ON SOCIETY

THE IMPACT OF SELF-MEDICATION ON SOCIETY

Higo José Neri da Silva Mateus Sávio Amorim Silva Keylla da Conceição Machado Kátia da Conceição Machado Jadielson da Silva Santos Larissa dos Santos Pessoa Manoela Carine Lima de Freitas

SUMMARY

Self-medication is a common practice in Brazil and around the world. Studies show that this activity can be practiced by purchasing medication without a prescription, sharing medication with other members of the family or social circle and using leftover prescriptions, reusing old prescriptions and failing to comply with professional prescriptions, prolonging or prematurely interrupting the dosage and the period of time indicated in the prescription. Its main objective is to analyze the risks of self-medication for society. To report what leads to this self-medication; to talk about self-medication and its effects; to demonstrate the need for correct medication for the population. The data will be collected using scientific databases: Latin American and Caribbean literature in health sciences - *LILACS,* national center for biotechnology information - PUBMED *virtual health library - BVS, SCIELO.* The papers will be analyzed at world, national and state level, and compared for greater relevance of the results, highlighting the impact of self-medication on society, analyzed in research. The consumption of medicines is related to advertising and marketing, which are widely used in the various media. This is why many people find information through the media.

Key words: Medication. Health. Self-medication. Drugs.

ABSTRACT

Self-medication is a common practice in Brazil and around the world. Studies indicate that this activity can be practiced when purchasing medication without a prescription, sharing medications with other members of the family or social circle and using leftover prescriptions, reusing old prescriptions and failing to comply with professional prescriptions, prolonging or prematurely interrupting the dosage and period time indicated in the prescription. Its main objective is to analyze the risks of self-medication for society. Report what leads to this self-medication; talking about self-medication and its effects; demonstrate the need for correct medication for the population. Data will be collected using scientific bases: Latin American and Caribbean literature in health sciences - LILACS, national center for biotechnology information - PUBMED virtual health library - VHL, SCIELO. Work at a global, national and state level will be analyzed; and compared for greater relevance of results. praising the impact of self-medication on society, analyzed in research. The consumption of medicines is related to advertising and marketing, widely used in various media. That's why many people find information through media outlets.

Keywords: Medicine. Health. Self-medication. Pharmacists.

SUMMARY

Self-medication is a common practice in Brazil and around the world. Studies indicate that this activity can be practiced by buying medicines without a prescription, sharing medicines with other members of the family or social circle and using leftover prescriptions, reusing old prescriptions and failing to comply with professional prescriptions, prolonging or prematurely interrupting the dosage and time period indicated in the prescription. Its main objective is to analyze the risks of self-medication for society. To inform about what leads to this self-medication; to talk about self-medication and its effects; to demonstrate the need for correct medication for the population. The data will be collected using scientific databases: Literatura Latinoamericana y del Caribe en Ciencias de la Salud - LILACS, Centro Nacional de Información Biotecnológica - Biblioteca Virtual en Salud PUBMED - BVS, SCIELO. Work at global, national and state level will be analyzed and compared to obtain greater relevance of the results. praising the impact of self-medication on society, analyzed in an investigation. The consumption of medicines is related to advertising and marketing, which are widely used in various media. That's why many people find information through the media.

Palabras clave: Medicine. Health Self-medication. Pharmacists.

INTRODUCTION

Self-medication is a common practice in Brazil and around the world. Studies show that this activity can be practiced by purchasing medication without a prescription, sharing medication with other members of the family or social circle and using leftover prescriptions, reusing old prescriptions and failing to comply with professional prescriptions, prolonging or prematurely interrupting the dosage and the period of time indicated in the prescription (FERRAZ, 2017).

In the context of human history, self-medication has been used since the beginning of human existence. During many phases of the evolution of history, we have always sought to develop various therapeutic forms to alleviate the symptoms presented during the onset of an illness, either through natural herbicides with curative purposes, homemade medicines, galenic mixtures, and also industrialized medicines (SESSO, 2017).

Drugs have a close relationship with health, from delaying the development of an illness to curing it. However, when used irrationally, they can cause a risk to an individual's state of health, intoxication or death. In current therapeutic treatment, drugs are seen as an important element, with a curative purpose, and to control pathologies, with great cost-effectiveness through rational use (OLIVEIRA, 2018).

Some of the conditions that favor the expansion of this practice in the world are political, cultural and economic, and it is seen as a serious public health problem. The huge increase in supply on the market means that the lay consumer becomes familiar with medicines. Allied to these conditions are other factors, such as the existence of gaps in health care and the difficulty of health services in underdeveloped countries (SARAN, 2020).

The WHO has reported that in Brazil drugs are sold in large quantities, approximately 30,000 a year. One possible reason for these figures is that pharmacies are seen as commercial outlets rather than health facilities. So how serious is self-medication in society?

Its main objective is to analyze the risks of self-medication for society. To report what leads to this self-medication; to talk about self-medication and its effects; to demonstrate the need for correct medication for the population.

METHODS

This is a qualitative study, with descriptive and explanatory objectives and a qualitative approach. Through scientific publications, this research seeks to describe its results, explaining their causes and effects. Its approach implies that everything carried out will be qualified and quantified in order to better demonstrate the results obtained by the research. Statistics will be used to better distribute and interpret the data (KAUARK, 2010).

All publications with data on the impact of self-medication on society, official World *Health Organization* (WHO) and governmental, from a given date (2019-2023) will be used.

Data will be collected using scientific databases: Latin American and Caribbean literature in health sciences - *LILACS,* National Center for Biotechnology Information - PUBMED, *Virtual Health Library - VHL, SCIELO.* The papers will be analyzed at world, national and state level; and compared for greater relevance of the results. highlighting the impact of self-medication on society, analyzed in research.

RESULTS

A total of 13 articles were selected from the scientific databases after applying the inclusion and exclusion criteria. The following databases were used: Latin American and Caribbean Health Sciences Literature (LILACS), *National Library of Medicine* (PUBMED), PERIODICALS, SCIENCE DIRECT, Virtual Health Library (BVS), *Scientific Electronic Library Online* (SCIELO), Cochrane Library, HighWire Press, Scopus and Elsevier. They were discussed in topic form.

DISCUSSION

2.1 Histories of pharmacy and medicines

It is clear that since the emergence of disease, man has always sought ways to find a cure. Ancient texts report the use of plants and substances of animal origin for curative purposes, dating back to the Paleolithic period or the age of chipped stone. The oldest known pharmaceutical document is a Sumerian tablet, made in the third millennium (2100 BC), containing fifteen medicinal recipes, discovered in Nippur. The most important papyrus in the history of Pharmacy is the Ebers papyrus written around 1500 BC, a kind of manual for students, which reveals medication secrets (SECOLI, 2018).

This veritable pharmacopoeia contains a wealth of information, 811 prescriptions and 700 remedies for various diseases, from snakebite to puerperal fever. Ancient Greece saw the beginning of modern medicine through the use of apothecaries, also known as apothéke, a word of Greek origin meaning a small box for storing drugs and used on trips made by doctors during health care (PEREIRA, 2017).

Until the 11th century, medicine and pharmacy were a single profession, but in 1240 AD, the Roman emperor Frederick II published the Magna Carta declaring pharmacy an independent profession. During the colonial period, the apothecary appeared in Brazil. In addition, apothecaries sold medicines and other products with a curative purpose, while the apothecary usually produced and administered the drug in front of the patient according to the prescription and the pharmacopoeia (BERTOLDI, 2016).

2.2 On self-medication

During the 1970s and 1980s, the ease of access to pharmaceuticals began to expand, since it is considered a component of health care that no diagnosis, prevention or treatment can be made without consulting a doctor or dentist. Quality of life linked to health is associated with the conditions in which human beings find themselves. Quality of life linked to health is the degree of importance that life should be classified and the functional complexities that can appear at any given time, such as illnesses, social conditions, perceptions, aggravated by political and economic issues in the health and treatment system (SARAN, 2020).

The influx of new drugs in recent years has led to a dramatic improvement in drug therapy, but it has also created problems. Not the least of which is the expression used to refer to the combination of the overwhelming number of drugs, confusion over drug nomenclature and the situation of uncertainty associated with many of them... The doctor can help to remedy this situation by prescribing products by their non-commercial names

(OLIVEIRA, 2018).

Medicines are necessary and relevant products for humans, along with housing, nutrition and other factors that describe the health index. However, it has become controversial due to irrational use because its therapeutic function is associated with social and economic issues, not related to illness and health. Self-medication is characterized as any initiative by a patient or their guardian to purchase medicines without a prescription from a legally qualified professional (SESSO, 2017).

Another concept of self-medication is the act of consuming medication without a prescription. This occurs through the patient deciding which medication to use in order to cure, and minimize signs through health promotion. Since self-medication is widely inserted as a practice practiced by Brazilians, both due to the difficulty of accessing health services and by the less privileged classes in search of quick solutions to remedy pathologies in order to prevent their daily activities from being impeded (FERRAZ, 2017).

Toxicology is the science that studies the adverse consequences of chemical substances on the body and also describes the chance and probability of their occurrence. Toxic agents generally related to intoxication are anticholinesterases, salicylates, metaboglobin, carboxyhemoglobin, barbiturates, cocaine and paracetamol (PRADO, 2016).

Some of the situations related to self-medication are: using the wrong dosage, using medication for a non-corresponding pathology, disregarding the information on the package leaflet regarding contraindications, abusive dependence, drug interactions that lead to a worsening of the clinical condition. It is also worth noting that the elderly are the group most at risk, since they are the people who most polymedicate, due to need and physiological fragility, so cases of drug interaction in the elderly are frequent (DOMINGUES, 2018).

The level of schooling and information is linked to this practice, as is the ease of access to medicines in the health system. Brazil is an emerging country and is far from being classified as a developed country, since the reality is different, especially when compared to the consumption of drugs ifirst world countries. This is why there is an alarming rate of people who self-medicate in Brazil, coupled with investment from the pharmaceutical industry, which spares no effort to promote its products through marketing and drug advertisements (SECOLI, 2018).

Pharmacies are described as veritable supermarkets, producing a culture of unbridled consumption. Incorrect self-diagnosis during the practice of self-medication can lead to a more serious illness, or its concealment, which hinders the effectiveness of therapeutic treatment (FERRAZ, 2017).

2.3 Marketing and drug advertisements

The Vargas government approved and authorized radio broadcasting. Rádio Nacional was one of the most renowned stations in 1936, and at this time commercial advertisers were already working, as was the case with products from the Sidney Ross Laboratory. Sonrisal, Colírio Moura Brasil, Urodonal and Elixir de Inhame were advertised. Television in Brazil came about during the 50s. With the emergence ofelevision, which will become the most widely televised media, it has become easier to understand how to capture the information transmitted within the reach of several people (PRADO, 2016).

The consumption of medicines is linked to advertising and marketing, which are widely used in the various media. That's why many people find information through the media. Anvisa says that during the campaign there is an incentive to continue consuming medicines. In today's consumer society, medicine is conceived as a product that needs to be constantly updated and renewed in its presentation. This is coupled with science, which aims to guarantee the efficacy and safety of the product for the user. In addition, the symbolism of health strengthens consumption habits by presenting medicine to the consumer in a seductive and saleable way and not with the simple recovery and quality of health (OLIVEIRA, 2018).

Today, the internet is the greatest media invention, used by a large number of people. Through this means of communication there are ways of putting the commercial marketing of the drug industry into practice. Therefore, it can be inferred that self-medication is related to the ease of obtaining information through this media (DOMINGUES, 2018).

REFERENCES

1. FERRAZ FHRP, RODRIGUES CIS, GATTO GC, SÁ NM. Differences and inequalities in relation to access to renal replacement therapy in the BRICS countries. Ciênc Saúde Colet. 2017;22(7):2175-85.

2. SESSO RC, LOPES AA, THOMÉ FS, LUGON JR, MARTINS CT. Brazilian chronic dialysis survey 2016. J Bras Nefrol. 2017;39(3):261-6.

3. OLIVEIRA JGR, SILVA GB JR, VASCONCELOS JE FILHO. Chronic kidney disease: exploring new communication strategies for health promotion. Rev Bras Promoç Saúde. 2018;31(4):1-8.

4. MINISTRY OF HEALTH, Health Surveillance Secretariat. National Health Promotion Policy. 3rd ed. Brasília: Ministry of Health; 2010.

5. SARAN R, ROBINSON B, ABBOTT KC, BRAGG-GRESHAM J, CHEN X, GIPSON D, et al. US Renal Data System 2019 Annual Data Report: epidemiology of kidney disease in the United States. Am J Kidney Dis. 2020;75(suppl 1).

6. SECOLI SR, MARQUESINI EA, FABRETTI SC, CORONA LP, ROMANO-LIEBER NS. Self-medication practice trend among the Brazilian elderly between 2006 and 2010: SABE Study. Rev Bras Epidemiol. 2018;21(Suppl 2):E180007.

7. PEREIRA FGF, ARAÚJO MJP, PEREIRA CR, NASCIMENTO DS, GALIZA FT, BENÍCIO CDAV. Self-medication in active elderly people. J Nurs UFPE. 2017;11(12):4919-28.

8. BERTOLDI AD, PIZZOL TSD, RAMOS LR, MENGUE SS, LUIZA VL, Tavares NUL, et al. Sociodemographic profile of medicines users in Brazil: results from the 2014 PNAUM survey. Rev Saúde Pública. 2016;50(Suppl 2):5s.

9. PRADO MAMB, FRANSCISCO PMSB, BASTOS TF, BARROS MBA. Use of prescription drugs and self-medication among men. Rev Bras Epidemiol. 2016;19(3):596-608.

10. DOMINGUES PHF, GALVÃO TF, ANDRADE KRC, ARAÚJO PC, SILVA MT, PEREIRA MG. Prevalence and associated factors of self-medication in adults living in the Federal District, Brazil: a cross-sectional, population-based study. Epidemiol Serv Saúde. 2017;26(2):319-30.

CHAPTER 5

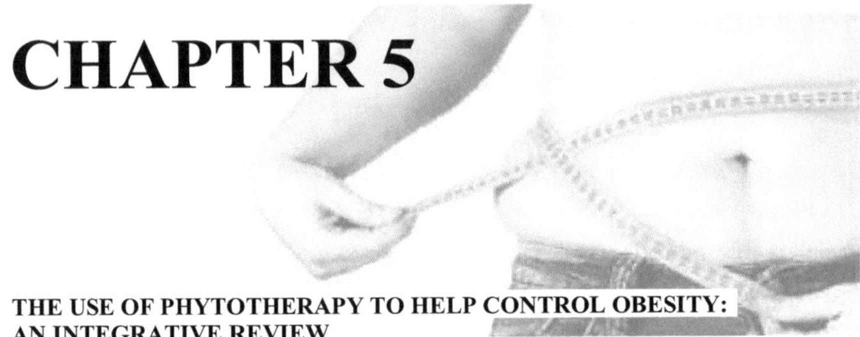

THE USE OF PHYTOTHERAPY TO HELP CONTROL OBESITY: AN INTEGRATIVE REVIEW

THE USE OF PHYTOTHERAPY DOES NOT HELP CONTROL OBESITY: INTEGRATIVE REVIEW

THE USE OF PHYTOTHERAPY DOES NOT HELP TO CONTROL OBESITY: INTEGRATIVE REVIEW

Larissa dos Santos Pessoa Higo José Neri da Silva Mateus Sávio Amorim Silva Keylla da Conceição Machado Kátia da Conceição Machado Jadielson da Silva Santos

Manoela Carine Lima de Freitas **ABSTRACT**

According to the World Health Organization (WHO), obesity is a modern pathology and one of the most rapidly developing diseases in recent years. Obesity and overweight are defined as an excessive or abnormal accumulation of fat that can affect health, with obese individuals being at greater risk of developing serious pathologies. The main objective is to demonstrate the importance of phytotherapy in combating obesity. Data will be collected using scientific databases: Latin American and Caribbean literature in health sciences - *LILACS,* national center for biotechnology information - PUBMED *virtual health library - BVS, SCIELO.* The studies will be analyzed at world, national and state level, and compared for greater relevance of the results, highlighting the importance of the use of herbal medicine in helping to control obesity, analyzed in research. The treatment of obesity can encompass a combination of procedures, such as medication, behavioral change training, surgical procedures and adherence to specific diets.

Key words: Medication. Health. Obesity. Drugs.

ABSTRACT

Obesity is a modern pathology, being one of the diseases with the greatest development in recent years, according to the World Health Organization (WHO). Obesity and overweight are defined as excessive or abnormal accumulation of fat that can affect health, placing obese individuals at greater risk of developing serious pathology. The main objective is to demonstrate the importance of phytotherapy to combat obesity. Data will be collected using scientific bases: Latin American and Caribbean literature in health sciences - LILACS, national center for biotechnology information - PUBMED virtual health library - VHL, SCIELO. Work at a global, national and state level will be analyzed; and compared for greater relevance of results. praising the importance of using herbal medicine to help control obesity, detailed in research. Obesity treatment may include a combination of procedures, such as medications, behavior change training, surgical procedures and adherence to specific diets.

Keywords: Medicine. Health. Obesity. Pharmacists.

SUMMARY

According to the World Health Organization (WHO), obesity is a modern pathology and one of the most rapidly developing diseases in recent years. Obesity and overweight are defined as an excessive or abnormal accumulation of fat that can affect health, putting obese people at greater risk of developing serious pathologies. The main objective is to demonstrate the importance of herbal medicine in the fight against obesity. The data will be collected using scientific databases: Literatura Latinoamericana y del Caribe en Ciencias de la Salud - LILACS, Centro Nacional de Información Biotecnológica - Biblioteca Virtual en Salud PUBMED - BVS, SCIELO. Work at global, national and state level will be analyzed and compared to obtain greater relevance of the results. Praise the importance of using medicinal herbs to help control obesity, as detailed in an investigation. The treatment of obesity can include a combination of procedures such as medication, training for behavior change, surgical procedures and adherence to specific diets.

Key words: Medicine. Health Obesity. Pharmacists.

INTRODUCTION

According to the World Health Organization (WHO), obesity is a modern pathology and one of the most rapidly developing diseases in recent years. Obesity and overweight are referred to as excessive or abnormal fat accumulation that can affect health, with obese individuals being at greater risk of developing serious pathologies (SOUZA et al., 2018).

Obesity and overweight in Brazil increase every year, reaching frightening numbers. In April 2017, the WHO reported data showing an increase in obesity in Brazil. According to the survey, one in five people in the country is overweight. The incidence of the condition rose from 11.8% in 2006 to 18.9% in 2016. Overweight is a key risk factor for chronic non-communicable diseases such as diabetes, hypertension, cardiovascular diseases and cancer, representing a serious public health problem (NÓBREGA NETO et al., 2017).

The three forms of treatment for weight control are medication, diet and exercise. Pharmacological treatment is used as a complementary therapy in conjunction with physical exercise and diet. Among the drugs that can be used in the weight loss process are herbal medicines (RODRIGUES DN; RODRIGUES DF, 2017).

However, knowledge and use of herbal medicines for the treatment of obesity is extremely important. Various parts can be used, such as leaves, stems, flowers, roots and fruits, which have both pharmacological and medicinal actions, as well as technical, food or cosmetic adjuvants (WEISHEIMER et al., 2015).

Phytotherapy is a sector that is growing and developing. One of the reasons for this increase is that people want to return to a more natural way dlife and are convinced that natural products are safe and healthy. This is what has brought these herbal medicines to the fore. So how important is the use of herbal medicine in obesity?

Phytotherapy is a sector that is growing and developing. One of the reasons for this increase is that people want to return to a more natural way dlife and are convinced that natural products are safe and healthy. This is what has brought these herbal medicines to the fore. So how important is the use of herbal medicine in obesity?

The main objective is to demonstrate the importance of herbal medicine in combating obesity. Evaluate the benefits of phytotherapy; evaluate its benefits for obesity; analyze the use of phytotherapy and its cost.

METHODS

This is a qualitative study, with descriptive and explanatory objectives and a qualitative approach. Through scientific publications, this research seeks to describe its results, explaining their causes and effects. Its approach implies that everything carried out will be qualified and quantified in order to better demonstrate the results obtained by the research. Statistics will be used to better distribute and interpret the data (KAUARK, 2010).

All publications with data on the use of herbal medicine to help control obesity, official from the *world* health organization (who) and governmental, between a certain date (2019-2023) will be used.

Data will be collected using scientific databases: Latin American and Caribbean literature in health sciences - *LILACS,* National Center for Biotechnology Information - PUBMED, *Virtual Health Library - VHL, SCIELO.* The studies will be analyzed at world, national and state level; and compared for greater relevance of the results. highlighting the importance of the use of phytotherapy in helping to control obesity, analyzed in research.

This research will use all studies that report on the use of herbal medicine to help control obesity, published between 2019 and 2023, in English and Portuguese. All other studies that do not fit the proposed theme and publications in other languages not mentioned above will be excluded.

RESULTS

A total of 13 articles were selected from the scientific databases after applying the inclusion and exclusion criteria. The following databases were used: Latin American and Caribbean Health Sciences Literature (LILACS), *National Library of Medicine* (PUBMED), PERIODICALS, SCIENCE DIRECT, Virtual Health Library (BVS), *Scientific Electronic Library Online* (SCIELO), Cochrane Library, HighWire Press, Scopus and Elsevier. They were discussed in topic form.

DISCUSSION

2.1 OBESITY

Obesity is a chronic, progressive pathology characterized by the accumulation of adipose tissue due to an imbalance between excessive calorie consumption and energy expenditure. It is essential to distinguish obesity as a public health problem, which can be caused at any age and affects a large part of the population (ZAROS, 2018).

According to the WHO, obesity is one of the world's biggest public health problems. It is estimated that, by 2025, more than 700 million adults will be obese and 2.3 billion overweight; and around 75 million children will be overweight or obese worldwide. In Brazil, estimates show that more than 50% of people are overweight, i.e. in the overweight-obesity range, and children would be around 15% (MARQUES, 2018).

Obesity is more prevalent in women, and it is thought that approximately 30% of adult women close to the menopause suffer from this disease. In Brazil, this rate is as high as 12.5%. This condition is more serious to the world's health authorities because it is directly correlated with the development of cardiovascular pathologies, Diabetes Mellitus (DM), Systemic Arterial Hypertension (SAH), neoplasms such as colon, breast and endometrial cancer (ALVES, 2018).

The etiology of obesity is characterized as multifactorial and can be genetic in origin, but is especially due to a sedentary lifestyle and inadequate diet, causing an imbalance in the energy balance, i.e. the calories consumed are greater than those expended. In addition, hormonal, environmental, social and pathological factors stand out, the latter two sometimes associated with drug treatments contributing to the condition of obesity (RODRIGUES, 2017).

2.2 OBESITY TREATMENT

The treatment of obesity can encompass a combination of procedures, such as medication, behavioral change training, surgical procedures and adherence to specific diets. Among these alternatives, for people with a BMI over 40, or over 35 with comorbidities, bariatric surgery has been shown to be an effective intervention for short-term weight loss. However, reducing and maintaining body weight depends on acquiring and maintaining behavioral habits related to diet (SOUZA, 2018).

2.3 TREATMENT WITH HERBAL MEDICINES

Phytotherapy is becoming an attractive treatment for obesity, as its natural aspect, low cost, easy accessibility for the population and few side effects are elements that make herbal medicines increasingly popular. Due to the different ways in which these natural products have been marketed recently, quality, safety and guaranteed efficacy are essential if they are to be used correctly. In addition, proper nutrition and physical exercise must also be combined (ZAMBON, 2018).

Herbal medicines, with scientifically confirmed quality and efficacy and registered with an authorized federal agency, are considered acceptable alternatives for use in the therapeutic arsenal. Herbal medicines used for weight control act on the body as metabolism accelerators or appetite modulators, promoting a reduction in food intake, reducing serum cholesterol levels, as well as having antioxidant, lipolytic and diuretic effects. A wide variety of natural substances have been analyzed for their potential in the treatment of obesity. These are generally complex products with diverse constituents and different pharmacological and chemical characteristics (PESSOA, 2017).

Every day, people are looking for drugs to help them lose weight, and there are many that are recommended by people who have no knowledge of the subject. However, it is important to note that herbal medicines also affect the health of those who do not use them properly. Many of them have active ingredients with the ability to modify organic functions, as well as interfere with the effect of medicines when used simultaneously, because even though they are over-the-counter, it is essential for a health professional to inform and guide you, because the irrational use of herbal medicines must be prevented (LOVATO, 2018).

Currently, the vegetable plants Phaseolus vulgaris (Phaseolamine), Garcinia cambogia (Garcinia), Cammelia sinensis (Green tea), Hibiscus sabdariffa L. (Hibiscus), Phaseolus vulgares L. (White beans), Cynara scolymus (Artichoke) have been gaining ground in the country in complementary therapy for obesity. Their pharmaceutical formulas are presented as teas, capsules and tinctures (ALVES, 2018).

Garcinia - Garcinia cambogia Garcinia (Garcinia cambogia - Gc) is a fruit from India. Its rind has phytotherapeutic action because it contains hydroxycitric acid (HCA), which is a key player in the metabolism of fatty acids (FA) and carbohydrates, as well as inhibiting appetite (ARAÚJO, 2018).

Green tea - Cammelia sinensis Cammelia sinensis, popularly known as green tea, is a plant known worldwide. From the processing of this plant, different herbal products are acquired, thus, different types of teas are generically known, all of which are produced from the same plant, but differ in the way they are prepared and fermented: green tea, oolong tea, black tea and Indian tea (MARQUES, 2018).

Hibiscus - Hibiscus sabdariffa L. Hibiscus sabdariffa L. belongs to the Malvaceae family and is popularly known in Brazil as hibiscus, hibiscus, gooseberry, roselle, sour okra, azedinha. Many beneficial activities are attributed to hibiscus, such as its antioxidant effect, and it is used to treat high blood pressure, cholesterol, lower total lipid levels, gastrointestinal disorders, obesity and liver infections (VIEIRA, 2019).

White beans - Phaseolus vulgares L Beans (Phaseolus vulgares L) are a legume that is an important source of iron, protein and vitamins for individuals. Among the different types of bean, white beans stand out because they have a better protein quality than other beans. In addition, this type of bean has resistant starch, which helps with weight loss by increasing satiety, and contributes to lowering triglycerides, blood glucose and serum cholesterol (VERBINEN, 2018).

Artichoke - Cynara scolymus The artichoke (Cynara scolymus) is a plant grown in the Atlantic regions. It has choleretic, cholagogue, hepatostimulant, hypocholesterolemic and diuretic effects. The leaves are used, and its active ingredient is extracted from acid alcohols: malic, glyceric, glycolic, citric, lactic and succinic, methyl-acrylic; sesquiterpene a-yielding lactones: cinaratriol, geosheimine, cinaropicrine, dihydrocinaropicrine, cinarolidine, rossheimine, grosulfeimine and others. Its main indication is the treatment of obesity, when there is a simultaneous reduction in bile secretion (JESUS, 2017).

REFERENCES

SOUZA, Saul de Azevêdo et al. Adult obesity in nations: an analysis via beta regression models. Cadernos de Saúde Pública, v.34, n.8, 2018. Available at:< https:// www. scielosp.org/article/csp/2018.v34n8/e00161417/ >.

NÓBREGA NETO, Henrique de Medeiros. Medicinal plants as adjuncts in the treatment of obesity and associated morbidities. II Brazilian Congress of Health Sciences, 2017. Available at:< http://editorarealize.com.br/ revistas/ conbracis/ trabalhos/ TRABALHO _EV071_ MD4 _SA6 _ID 1860 _1505 2017 183 442 .pdf>.

RODRIGUES, Dhulia Nogueira; RODRIGUES, Debora Fernandes. Phytotherapy as an adjunct in the treatment of obesity. Brazilian Journal of Life Sciences, v. 5, n. 4, 2017. Available at: <http:// jornal . facul dade cienciasdavida .com. br/ index .php/RBCV/article/view/379>.

WEISHEIMER, Naiana et al. Phytotherapy as a therapeutic alternative in the fight against obesity. Revista de Ciências da Saúde Nova Esperança, v.13, n.1, 2015. Available at:< http:// www. facene.com.br/wp-content/uploads/2010/11/Fitoterapiacomo- alternativa-PRONTO.pdf >.

ALVES, Cristiano Alberto de Lima. Bibliographic review on the characterization of herbal medicines with potential for use in weight loss. 2018. 39f. Monograph (Degree in Pharmacy) - Faculty of Health Sciences, University of Brasília. Brasília. Available at:<

http://bdm.unb.br/ bitstream/ 10483/21234/1/2018_ CristianoAlbertoDeLimaAlves_tcc.pdf>.

ARAÚJO, Raquel Pessoa; MORAIS, Selene Maia. Medicinal plants for obesity control. Temas em Saúde, João Pessoa, v.18, n.2, 2018. Available at:< http://temasemsaude.com/wp-content/uploads/2018/07/18217.pdf>.

BRITO, Janaina Vidal Bezerra et al. Main herbal medicines used in the treatment of obesity, sold in a compounding pharmacy. Brazilian Journal of Surgery and Clinical Research - BJSCR, v. 27, n.1, 2019. Available at:< https://www.mastereditora. com.br/ periodico/ 20190607_201754.pdf>.

CONCEIÇÃO, Francileine Rodrigues et al. Complementary therapy: The commercialization of herbal medicines for weight control in a municipality in Maranhão. REAS, Acervo Saúde Electronic Journal, 2018. Available at:< https://www. acervo saude .com.br/doc/REAS188.pdf>.

JESUS, Cleidymar Menezes et al. Treatment of obesity through dietary re-education associated with the use of herbal medicines. Multidisciplinary Journal of the Northeast of Minas Gerais - Unipac, 2017. Available at:< http://www.unipacto.com.br/revista-multi disciplinar/arquivos _pdf_revista/ revista 2017_1/26.pdf>.

LOVATO, Frederico et al. Centesimal composition and mineral content of different biorfortified bean cultivars (Phaseolus vulgaris L.). Brazilian Journal of Food Technology, Campinas, v. 21, 2018. Available at:< http://www.scielo.br/pdf/bjft/ v21/ 1981-6723-bjft-21-e2017068.pdf >.

MARQUES, Dalília Pereira et al. Nutrition and phytotherapy as an aid in the treatment of obesity. Revela, ed. 22, 2018. Available at:< http://fals.com.br/revela/ed22/ ED22_T7.pdf>.

PESSOA, Érika Vicência Monteiro; SOUSA, Francisco Das Chagas Araújo. Effect of garcinia cambogia administration on weight reduction. Revista Ciências e Saberes FAECEMA, v.3, n.2, 2017. Available at:< http://www.facema.edu.br/ojs/ index.php/ReOnFacema/article/view/199/118>.

VERBINEN, A.; OLIVEIRA, V. B. The use of Garcinia cambogia as an adjunct in the treatment of obesity. Visão Acadêmica, Curitiba, v.19 n.3, 2018. Available at:< https://revistas. ufpr.br/ academica/article/download/ 59541/ 37417>.

VIEIRA, Adna Rosanny dos Reis; MEDEIROS, Priscilla Ramos Mortate da Silva. The use of herbal medicines in the treatment of obesity. Revista Cientifica da Escola Estadual de Saúde Pública de Goiás "Cândido Santiago", v.5, n.1, 2019. Available at:< www.revista.esap.go. gov.br/ index. php/resap/ article/ down load /111/128/>.

ZAMBON, Camila Pereira et al. The use of herbal medicines in the weight loss process in pharmacy students at the Faculty of Education and Environment - FAEMA. Revista Cientifica FAEMA, v.9, 2018. Available at:< http://www.faema.edu.br/revistas/index.php/Revista-FAEMA/article/ view/ rcf. v9ied esp.621/538>.

ZAROS, Karin Juliana Bitencourt. Off-label use of obesity drugs. Bulletin of the Center for Information on Medicines, ed. 2, 2018. Available at:< https://crf-pr.org.br/uploads/revista/ 33657/ CeW0q ho1Z WuSJ g2 f4Ioml1hrF99F2Etv.pdf>.

CHAPTER 6

THE IMPORTANCE OF GENERIC MEDICINES FOR SOCIETY

GENERIC MEDICINES ARE IMPORTANT FOR SOCIETY

GENERIC DRUGS ARE IMPORTANT FOR SOCIETY

Larissa dos Santos Pessoa Higo José Neri da Silva Mateus Sávio Amorim Silva Keylla da Conceição Machado Kátia da Conceição Machado Jadielson da Silva Santos

SUMMARY

The pharmaceutical formulation industry in Brazil is represented by a sector with an annual turnover of more than three billion dollars, making it one of the ten largest markets in the world. Assess the importance of generic drugs for society. Assess their financial benefits; evaluate existing projects and disclosures; analyze how their market works. The data will be collected using scientific databases: Latin American and Caribbean literature in health sciences - *LILACS,* national center for biotechnology information - PUBMED *virtual health library - BVS, SCIELO.* It is clear that the production of generic drugs is a trend that is being observed in developed countries, and the WHO recommends its implementation as the backbone of a policy for developing countries. We believe that, for the Brazilian market, generic drugs also represent a concrete alternative, provided that a series of concepts and procedures are defined and implemented by the different players involved in the process. The mere existence of products with generic names is not enough to establish the necessary competitiveness or influence market prices.

Key words: Medication. Health. ADHD. Drugs.

ABSTRACT

The pharmaceutical formulation industry in Brazil is represented by a sector that generates more than three billion dollars annually, making it one of the ten largest markets in the world. Assess the importance of generic medicines for society. Assess your financial benefits; evaluate existing projects and disclosures; analyze how your market works. Data will be collected using scientific bases: Latin American and Caribbean literature in health sciences - LILACS, national center for biotechnology information - PUBMED virtual health library - VHL, SCIELO. It is clear that the production of generic medicines represents a trend that is observed both in developed countries, and the WHO also recommends its implementation as the backbone of a policy for developing countries. We believe that, for the Brazilian market, generic medicines also represent a concrete alternative, as long as a series of concepts and procedures are defined and implemented by the different actors involved in the process. The simple existence of products with a generic name is not enough to establish competitiveness or influence market prices.

Keywords: Medicine. Health. ADHD. Pharmacists.

SUMMARY

The pharmaceutical formulations industry in Brazil is represented by a sector that generates more than three billion dollars a year, making it one of the ten largest markets in the world. Valuing the importance of generic medicines for society. Evaluate their financial benefits; evaluate existing projects and disclosures; analyze how your market works. The data will be collected using scientific databases: Literatura Latinoamericana y del Caribe en Ciencias de la Salud - LILACS, Centro Nacional de Información

Biotecnológica - Biblioteca Virtual en Salud PUBMED.
- BVS, SCIELO. It is clear that the production of generic medicines represents a trend observed in developed countries, and the WHO also recommends its implementation as the backbone of a policy for developing countries. We believe that, for the Brazilian market, generic drugs also represent a concrete alternative, provided that a series of concepts and procedures are defined and implemented by the different players involved in the process. The mere existence of products with a generic name is not enough to establish competitiveness or influence market prices.

Key words: Medicine. ADHD Health. Pharmacists.

INTRODUCTION

The pharmaceutical formulation industry in Brazil represents an annual turnover of more than three billion dollars, and is one of the ten largest markets in the world. With a low per capita consumption, it has a perverse distribution, considering that 23% of the population consumes 60% of production (DUNNE, 2015).

The government market represents around 35% of the total market. Our dependence is evident when we see that multinational companies are responsible for 75 to 85% of annual sales in Brazil. The situation becomes more serious when we see, along with a growing process of denationalization of the private sector, government action that does not strengthen state production laboratories (COELHO, 2020).

Brazil accounts for around 3.2% of the world market. The Brazilian industrial park in the fine chemicals complex has a measurable installed capacity of 500,000 tons per year. The situation observed in national companies is the use cfechnologies developed abroad, while multinational companies import the technology applied in their production and sales processes from their headquarters (GOMES, 2017).

According to a survey carried out by Codetec, raw materials produced domestically by national companies account for less than 10% of the total value of production. Our external dependence is clear and can be analyzed in conjunction with the issue of market oligopolization. A striking difference between the large multinational companies and our

Brazilian industries is that the former seek to verticalize their production, acting in all technological stages, including research, development of raw materials, formulation and marketing, while the majority of national companies only develop the pharmaceutical formulation stage, maintaining their dependence on the acquisition of raw materials (MARTICH, 2013).

The discussion of generic drugs, their global insertion and their evaluation as an alternative for the Brazilian market, is associated with a reflection on our healthcare model, as well as the market characteristics of the pharmaceutical industry in Brazil and worldwide. This discussion has to take into account the very conceptualization of medicines as health inputs or as goods aimed exclusively at profit. So what is the importance of generics for society?

Assess the importance of generic drugs for society. Assess their financial benefits; evaluate existing projects and disclosures; analyze how their market works.

METHODS

It is a qualitative study with descriptive and explanatory objectives and a qualitative approach. This study attempts to describe its results and explain their causes and effects through scientific publications. Its approach means that everything carried out will be qualified and quantified in order to better demonstrate the results obtained in the research. Statistics will be used to better distribute and interpret the data (KAUARK, 2010).
Articles will be used according to the proposed theme: the importance of generic drugs for society, official World *Health Organization* (WHO) and governmental articles, from a given date (2019-2023).
Data will be collected using the following scientific databases: Latin American and Caribbean Health Sciences Literature - *LILACS,* National Center for Biotechnology Information - PUBMED, *Virtual Health Library - VHL, SCIELO.* The data will be used according to the inclusion criteria proposed below.

RESULTS

A total of 13 articles were selected from the scientific databases after applying the inclusion and exclusion criteria. The following databases were used: Latin American and Caribbean Health Sciences Literature (LILACS), *National Library of Medicine* (PUBMED), PERIODICALS, SCIENCE DIRECT, Virtual Health Library (BVS), *Scientific Electronic Library Online* (SCIELO), Cochrane Library, HighWire Press, Scopus and Elsevier. They were discussed in topic form.

DISCUSSION

2.1 AN ALTERNATIVE FOR THE BRAZILIAN MARKET

It is clear that the production of generic medicines is a trend that is being observed in developed countries, and the WHO recommends its implementation as the backbone of a policy for developing countries. We believe that, for the Brazilian market, generic drugs also represent a concrete alternative, provided that a series of concepts and procedures are defined and implemented by the different players involved in the process. The mere existence of products with generic names is not enough to establish the necessary competitiveness or influence market prices (NIELSON, 2018).

A clear government policy needs to be established, including agreement mechanisms with the industry, commitment from the various categories of professionals involved, support from scientific society and health organizations, and all the necessary complementary legal framework. A number of concepts need to be clarified with regard to generic drugs and the Brazilian market. The multinational industries in Brazil have criticized and restricted the generics decree, claiming that replacing or prescribing generic drugs will lead to problems with the quality of the drugs. This criticism applies to similarity registrations. However, it is clear that the issue of monitoring and ensuring the quality of products circulating on the market is a crucial point in the implementation of a generic drug policy and must be taken up as a government action (DE AMORIM, 2020).

Another issue to clarify is the differentiation between "generic drugs" and the generic name of products already on the market. In this sense, we looked at the concepts of interchangeability, bioequivalence and bioavailability (COELHO, 2020).

2.2 THE PHARMACEUTICAL ASSISTANCE PROGRAM AND DECREE 793: ADVANCES AND OBSTACLES

As a result of the political conditions at the time, in accordance with WHO recommendations and based on the experience of other countries, decree 793, published in the Official Gazette of 6/4/93 and included in the Pharmaceutical Assistance Program drawn up by the Ministry of Health, presents the following advances in relation to the country's medicines policy: 1. determines the emphasis on the generic name of medicines over brand names; 2. also requires the presence of pharmacists in pharmacies, which only reiterates existing legislation. It also requires prescriptions to be made under the generic name, while it does not prohibit the use of fantasy brands; 3. It obliges pharmacists to be present in pharmacies, which only reiterates legislation that already exists in Brazil, as well as being routine practice in most countries; 4. It allows the packaging of medicines to be split up, as long as the original quality and therapeutic efficacy are guaranteed (CRUZ, 2021).

A series of obstacles have hindered the effective implementation of the decree, including numerous lawsuits, pressure from diplomatic representations, the weaknesses of the current national health surveillance system and the failure to implement actions at federal level, such as widely publicizing the correlation between generic names and brand names (MONTEIRO, 2016).

2.3 PERSPECTIVES AND PROPOSALS: NECESSARY ACTIONS

The effective implementation of a generic drug policy should be seen as an alternative for the Brazilian market, considering that the experience of other countries has shown that it effectively reduces prices by breaking the monopoly of brands and providing options for the population. However, a series of government actions are needed to ensure the quality and equivalence of licensed products. The difficulties in implementing decree 793/93 have shown that there are conflicts between the social interests of health policies and the commercial interests of pharmaceutical companies. At the same time as relationship mechanisms are agreed upon, the state's regulatory power must be exercised to the full and within the margins that our legislation establishes. A generic drug policy proposal must be a sectoral action, involving other ministries and other spheres of government, as well as society (DE OLIVEIRA, 2018).

As long as it is taken on with government political backing, the following points represent issues that need to be addressed in an integrated manner in order to implement a program of this type: 1. Review of the registration of licensed drugs, differentiating between those that are actually circulating on the market. 2. Analysis of registered products by therapeutic group, with identification of the innovative product and its respective dynamic drug analysis. 3) Establishment of bioequivalence and bioavailability requirements, with the list of tests to be carried out and their in vitro equivalence, to be determined by Ministerial Order. 4) Setting up and certifying the infrastructure at the National Institute for Quality Control in Health, capable of ensuring the necessary technical support and analysis capacity. 5) Immediate launch of regular inspection programs for industries, with an emphasis on Good Manufacturing Practices (GMP) and verification of quality control laboratories. 6) Establishment of reference price policies for medicines and a register of companies applying to produce generic medicines, with clear mechanisms for government-company coordination. 7. complementary actions, including the effective implementation of Decree 793, the strengthening of state laboratories, the establishment of auxiliary quality control laboratories, as well as the necessary legal framework and instruments (GUTTIER, 2016).

REFERENCES

COELHO, A. F., et al. Patient acceptance of generic drugs: a literature review. Rev. Saúde Viva Multidisciplinar da AJES, 3 (4). 2020.

CRUZ, A. F. P., et al. Factors associated with the acceptance of generic drugs by the population. Research, Society and Development, 10 (10), 1-8. 2021.

GOMES, L. S. S. Analysis of the knowledge and acceptance of generic drugs by health professionals at the Santa Casa de Misericórdia in the municipality dCachoeira, Bahia. Course Conclusion Work - Pharmacy Course - Maria Milza College, Governador Mangabeira, 1-87. 2017.

GUTTIER, M. C., et al. Perception, knowledge and use of generic drugs in Southern Brazil: what changed between 2002 and 2012? Cad. de Saúde Pública, 32 (7). 2016.

MARTICH, E. V. Generic drug policy and the pharmaceutical market in Argentina and Brazil. Sciences in Public Health, 8 (7). 2013.

MONTEIRO, C. N., et al. Use of generic drugs in the city of São Paulo in 2003: a population-based study. Epidemiol. Serv. Saúde, 35 (2). 2016.

DAVE, Chintan V. et al. High generic drug prices and market competition: a retrospective cohort study. Annals of internal medicine, v. 167, n. 3, p. 145-1

DE AMORIM RODRIGUES, Larice et al. Generic drugs in the last 20 years and consumer perception. Revista Saúde dos Vales; ISSN: 2674-8584 v.1, n.1. 2020.

DE OLIVEIRA LEMES, Erick et al. History of Generic Medicines in Brazil. Ensaios e Ciência C Biológicas Agrárias e da Saúde, v. 22, n. 2, p. 119-123, 2018.

DUNNE, Suzanne S.; DUNNE, Colum P. What do people really think of generic medicines? A systematic review and critical appraisal of literature on stakeholder perceptions of generic drugs. BMC medicine, v. 13, n. 1, p. 1-27, 2015.

NIELSON, Sylvia Escher de Oliveira et al. The importance of generic drugs in brazil. Revista de Trabalhos Acadêmicos-Universo-Goiânia, n. 4, 2018.

CHAPTER 7

NATURAL MEDICINE AS AN ALLY IN THE TREATMENT OF CHRONIC PAIN IN FIBROMYALGIA PATIENTS

NATURAL MEDICINE AS AN ALLY IN THE TREATMENT OF CHRONIC PAIN IN PATIENTS WITH FIBROMYALGIA

NATURAL MEDICINE AS AN ALLY IN THE TREATMENT OF CHRONIC PAIN IN FIBROMYALGIA PATIENTS

Kelly Maria Rêgo da Silva Manoela Carine Lima de Freitas
Michelle Diana Leal Pinheiro Matos Mac Dave Cardoso Ribeiro Matos Silva
Ricardo de Araújo
Eneas Costa Junior
Dênis Rômulo Leite Furtado

SUMMARY

Fibromyalgia is a chronic disease that unfortunately still has no origin and no cure. Around 2% to 3% of the world's population has the disease, which is more prevalent in women. This study aims to highlight and describe the need to explore integrative and complementary practices with an emphasis on medicinal plants and herbal medicines. Data will be collected using the following scientific databases: Latin American and Caribbean Health Sciences Literature - *LILACS,* National Center for Biotechnology

Information - *PUBMED, Virtual Health Library - VHL, SCIELO.* In 2010, new criteria were introduced by the *American College of Rheumatology*, requiring a search for points to check the severity of symptoms and the pain index. Other symptoms observed are: tendency to tiredness, psychological changes, joint swelling, headache and irritable bowel syndrome.

Key words: Medication. Health. Fibromyalgia. Drugs.

ABSTRACT

Fibromyalgia is a chronic disease that unfortunately has no origin and no cure. Around 2% to 3% of the world population has the disease, more predominantly in women. This study aims to highlight and describe the need to explore integrative and complementary practices with an emphasis on medicinal plants and herbal medicines. Data will be collected using scientific bases: Latin American and Caribbean Literature in Health Sciences - LILACS, National Center for Biotechnology Information - PUBMED, Virtual Health Library - VHL, SCIELO. In 2010, new criteria were created by the American College of Rheumatology and it was necessary to search for points to check the severity of symptoms and the pain index. Other symptoms observed are: tendency to tiredness, psychological changes, feeling of joint swelling, headache and irritable bowel syndrome.

Keywords: Medicine. Health. Fibromyalgia. Pharmacists.

SUMMARY

Fibromyalgia is a chronic illness that unfortunately has no origin or cure. Around 2% to 3% of the world's population suffers from the illness, predominantly in women. This study aims to highlight and describe the need to explore integrative and complementary practices with an emphasis on medicinal plants and medicinal herbs. The data will be collected from scientific databases: Literatura Latinoamericana y del Caribe en Ciencias de la Salud - LILACS, Centro Nacional de Información Biotecnológica - PUBMED, Biblioteca Virtual en Salud - BVS, SCIELO. In 2010, the American College of

Rheumatology created new criteria and it was necessary to look for points to verify the severity of the symptoms and the pain index. Other symptoms observed are: a tendency to tiredness, psychological changes, a feeling of swelling in the joints, headaches and irritable bowel syndrome.

Key words: Medicine. Health. Fibromyalgia. Pharmacists.

INTRODUCTION

Fibromyalgia is a chronic disease that unfortunately still has no origin and no cure. Around 2% to 3% of the world's population has the disease, which is more prevalent in women (HOLZER et al., 2021).

The disease consists of chronic central pain and somatic hypersensitivity. The quality of life of sufferers is an important part to be analyzed, as it has a high cost. The nervous system is very important in this disease and its alterations directly affect patients ESTÉVEZ-LÓPEZ et al., 2021).

Pharmacological therapy has been effective for a short period of time and is always accompanied by considerable side effects. As a result, there is a great need for alternative or complementary therapy, where of the existing forms of treatment, some phytotherapics and medicinal plants are the ones that have the most evidence for treating this pathology, thus encompassing a change in lifestyle and non-pharmacological and pharmacological interventions with the main objective of relieving pain and improving the quality of life of fibromyalgia patients. Over time, medicinal plants have been defined as those administered to humans or animals by some means and in a pharmaceutical form that has a therapeutic effect, and are considered the raw material for the manufacture of herbal medicines. The use of this activity has been present in humanity since the beginning, being one of the oldest practices known, dating back to around 8,500 B.C. and continues to be used to this day because it is easily accessible and relatively inexpensive (BELLATO et al., 2021).

Phytotherapy studies the application of plants or parts of them for therapeutic resources for some diseases, such as the use of herbal medicines acquired from a plant and which can be presented in various pharmaceutical forms such as teas, solutions, tablets and others. Around 80% of the population uses or has used this therapy as an alternative to medical treatment (FERRAN et al., 2021).

The use of medicinal plants in fibromyalgia has shown formidable therapeutic activities. Some plants have already shown efficacy in association with other synthetic drugs, thus verifying the comparable effectiveness of both for the treatment of the condition. Other medicinal plants have shown a reduction in associated symptoms such as anxiety, depression and an anti-inflammatory effect, improving chronic pain and reducing inflammation. However, fibromyalgia is a multidimensional disorder, so the use of combined therapy is necessary to improve the overall clinical condition of the patient affected by the disease. So here's the problem: Is there a herbal treatment that can treat fibromyalgia and thus avoid the possible side effects of other drugs?

This study aims to highlight and describe the need to explore integrative and complementary practices with an emphasis on medicinal plants and herbal medicines. To help patients with fibromyalgia; to reduce their symptoms; to improve the quality of life of those suffering from this disease.

METHODS

This is a qualitative study, with descriptive and explanatory objectives and a qualitative approach. Through scientific publications, this research seeks to describe its results, explaining their causes and effects. Its approach implies that everything carried out will be qualified and quantified in order to better demonstrate the results obtained by the research. Statistics will be used to better distribute and interpret the data (KAUARK, 2010).

All publications with data on natural medicine as an ally in the treatment of chronic pain in patients with fibromyalgia, scientific, official *World Health Organization* (WHO) and government publications, between a certain date (2018-2023) will be used.

Data will be collected using the following scientific databases: Latin American and

Caribbean Health Sciences Literature - *LILACS,* National Center for Biotechnology Information - *PUBMED, Virtual Health Library - VHL, SCIELO.*

Studies at world, national and state level will be analyzed and compared for greater relevance of the results. Praising natural medicine as an ally in the treatment of chronic pain in patients with fibromyalgia, analyzed in research.

RESULTS

A total of 13 articles were selected from the scientific databases after applying the inclusion and exclusion criteria. The following databases were used: Latin American and Caribbean Health Sciences Literature (LILACS), *National Library of Medicine* (PUBMED), PERIODICALS, SCIENCE DIRECT, Virtual Health Library (BVS), *Scientific Electronic Library Online* (SCIELO), Cochrane Library, HighWire Press, Scopus and Elsevier. They were discussed in topic form.

DISCUSSION

3.1 Fibromyalgia its origin and classification

Fibromyalgia is a chronic disease, which causes chronic skeletal muscle pain in general and great sensitivity in various areas of the body with persistent fatigue, muscle weakness, changes in sleep, coexistence with symptoms such as depression and anxiety (ESTÉVEZ-LÓPEZ et al., 2021).

The diagnostic criteria for the disease are established by the *American College of Rheumatology* (ACR) (in 1990) and are: pain in the body for more than three months, in various parts of the body with at least 11 to 18 points pressed (PERNAMBUCO et al., 2021).

In 2010, new criteria were introduced by the *American College of Rheumatology*, requiring the search for points to check the severity of symptoms and the pain index. Other symptoms observed are: tendency to fatigue, psychological changes, joint swelling, headache and irritable bowel syndrome (TOPRAK et al., 2021).

The pain varies over time, but never disappears completely. In the morning the pain is more intense, also with stress and anxiety. This has an impact on patients' daily lives (PASQUAL et al., 2021).

This pain in patients is related to the central nervous system, which also has a difference in stimuli. It is also linked to other alterations such as chronic fatigue syndrome or irritable bowel syndrome (RODRÍGUEZ et al., 2021).

Muller in 2007 classified the disease into four types: idiopathic, related to chronic diseases, fibromyalgia in patients with psychopathological illnesses (RIZZI et al., 2021).

Type one is made up of sufferers with extreme sensitivity to pain and a differential psychopathological profile. Type two is related to chronic diseases such as rheumatology and includes systemic diseases correlated with degeneration of musculoskeletal structures at a specific site (FERRAN et al., 2021).

Type three are patients with the disease and psychopathological problems (with a high degree of anxiety and depression) at a high level, increasing the pain. However, type four is called simulated fibromyalgia and is a syndrome of any pathologically defined nature, evidently proven by tests (BENNETT et al., 2021).

3.2 Pathophysiology and clinical manifestations

Even after much research, there is still no specific cause for the disease. However, this new research has made new advances, especially in terms of the possible origin of the disease. Recent research shows that there is biochemical, immunoregulatory and metabolic differentiation (BELLATO et al., 2021)

One of these biochemical variations is a reduction in serotonin, lower levels of tryptophan and 5-hydroxyindole acetic acid. There is also a 2 to 3-fold increase in substance P in the CSF. This neurotransmitter increases pain levels (GUMÀ-URIEL et al., 2016).

Another alteration observed is a dysfunction in the hypothalamic-pituitary-adrenal (H-H-A) axis and the locus coeruleus-norepinephrine (LCNE) axis, these axes are important components for the adaptive response to stress, these are stimulated by corticotropin-releasing hormone (HLC) (MÜLLER et al., 2021).

3.3 Alternative medicine for fibromyalgia

Alternative and complementary medicine has been much sought after by the population in recent years, especially among individuals with fibromyalgia, in which conventional therapy alone has shown limited benefits and which requires multidisciplinary treatment. In 1997, in a telephone survey of 2,055 people in the USA, 42% of them reported using some kind of alternative and/or complementary medicine in the year prior to the study. These included: medicinal herbs, multivitamins, massages, self-help groups, homemade formulations, religiosity and homeopathy, both in the prevention and treatment of specific illnesses (BARBOSA, COSTA, ALFENAS, PAULA & MININ, 2021).

In the same year, researchers examined the frequency of search and the factors that led 111 fibromyalgia patients to seek alternative and complementary medicine. They concluded that, in this group of patients, the intensity of pain and disability were the main factors leading a fibromyalgia patient to seek out this type of therapy. Another group conducted a study from February to July 2003 to verify the frequency and type of alternative and complementary medicine used in a tertiary fibromyalgia treatment center. Of the 289 patients who took part in the survey (263 women and 26 men), 98% reported using some kind of alternative and complementary therapy, and the ten most frequently mentioned were: exercise (48%), treatment through prayer (45%), massage therapy (44%), chiropractic (37%); use of vitamins C (35%) and E (31%), magnesium (29%), B complex (25%), green tea (24%) and weight loss programs (20%). Fifty-one percent of patients reported using one or more medicinal herbs or dietary supplements, and ginseng was reported by 8% of patients of all ages, mainly between 18 and 64 (ZHANG et al., 2021).

Although non-pharmacological treatments such as exercise and cognitive behavioral therapy are sometimes considered a form of alternative and complementary medicine, the National Institutes of Health (NIH) does not classify them as such. Historically, alternative and complementary medicine was defined as medical interventions not routinely prescribed by Western medical practitioners and not widely practiced in medical schools. The NIH classifies this type of medical practice into five groups: 1) alternative medicine: traditional Chinese medicine (including acupuncture), naturopathic medicine, ayurvedic medicine or homeopathy; 2) biologically based therapies, including herbal medicine, dietary supplementation and individual biological treatment - the latter not accepted by the FDA; 3) energy therapies, such as Reike, therapeutic touch and magnetic therapy, among others; 4) systems based on body manipulation: chiropractic, osteopathy and massage; 5) body-mind interventions, such as meditation, relaxation, biofeedback and hypnotherapy (SATOKARI et al., 2021; FRANCINO, 2021).

In alternative and complementary medicine, of the forms of treatment described above for fibromyalgia, with the exception of acupuncture, some herbal medicines, nutritional supplements and massages, the data in the literature showed a low level of evidence for the other types of therapies. According to Ernst,60 there is a trend towards positive results with homeopathy, but this data is insufficient to indicate its use (GAVANSKI, BARATTO & GATTI, 2021).

3.4 Diet, nutritional supplements and herbal medicine

Several authors have reported the beneficial effects of diet on the symptoms of rheumatological diseases, especially vegetarian diets. Researchers have studied the role of diet in the improvement of patients with fibromyalgia. The first carried out a study with 12 patients who received a mixture of ascorbic acid and broccoli and obtained a reduction in pain and quality of life parameters. The second evaluated the efficacy of a strictly vegetarian diet, concluding that it was beneficial, albeit for a short period. Both were open, non-randomized studies, requiring larger population groups and double-blind studies (COHEN et al., 2021).

Another study observed an improvement in various fibromyalgia monitoring parameters (pain, sleep, fatigue and quality of life) in 19 out of 30 patients who received an exclusive vegetarian diet for 7 months. However, this study had restrictions with regard to its design (non-controlled and open), in addition to the fact that all the patients maintained conventional treatment during the course of the work (CABEZAS et al., 2021).

S-adenosyl-L-methionine (SAMe) is one of the 25 most consumed dietary supplements in the USA. It has antidepressant, anti-inflammatory and analgesic properties. It demonstrated a significant improvement in the duration of morning stiffness, pain at rest, fatigue and overall disease activity, using a dose of 800 mg/day orally versus placebo for 6 weeks in 44 fibromyalgia patients. However, it was not well accepted due to the high incidence of side effects, and its effect on tender points, muscle strength and mood was no different from the control group (STILLING et al., 2021).

An herb considered to be a dietary supplement, Chorella pyrenoidosa (green, unicellular algae, rich in proteins, vitamins and mineral salts) has been shown to relieve some of the symptoms of fibromyalgia, especially a reduction in the number of tender points in two studies: an open study with 18 patients, and a randomized, double-blind, controlled study involving 37 individuals. Both studies were carried out by the same group, prompting the need to carry out more studies, with large samples and better design, which can prove these results by other study groups (CARABOTTI et al., 2021).

A randomized, controlled, double-blind study with Hypericum perfuratum and amitriptyline was carried out by the Rheumatology Discipline of the Federal University of São Paulo, with the aim of studying the efficacy and tolerability of H. perfuratum in the treatment of patients with fibromyalgia, based on the antidepressant properties of this plant. Seventy-nine patients randomized in a 1:1 ratio took part in the study. At the end of 12 weeks of treatment, both groups had improved significantly, compared to baseline, in relation to the visual analog scale of pain and the Fibromyalgia impact questionnaire (FIQ), with no differences between the groups. The authors concluded that, in this study, H. perfuratum and amitriptyline were effective in treating patients with fibromyalgia, with no differences between the two groups (HOLZER et al., 2021).

A cannabinoid phytodrug (nabilone), a selective antagonist of the serotonin receptor (5-HT3), was studied in a double-blind, placebo-controlled manner in 40 patients with fibromyalgia. Using nabilone orally at doses of 0.5 mg to 2 mg/day, there was a reduction in pain (visual analog scale for pain) and anxiety, suggesting the participation of this phytopharmaceutical as a probable adjuvant in the treatment of fibromyalgia. Panax ginseng C.A. Meyer is a herbal medicine that has been used in oriental medicine for hundreds of years, primarily to treat weakness and fatigue (OPIE et al., 2021).

Clinical studies evaluating the analgesic activities of P. ginseng are scarce in the literature. Recently, a randomized, double-blind, controlled clinical trial compared the action of P. ginseng root extract (100 mg/day) with amitriptyline (25 mg/day) and placebo in 38 women with bromyalgia for 12 weeks. Pain, fatigue, sleep and anxiety were assessed using the visual analog scale (VAS), the number of tender points and quality of life using the quality of life impact questionnaire (FIQ). In this study, P. ginseng was able to improve all the parameters assessed in relation to the baseline period, but was no different from placebo or amitriptyline, and the latter was superior to placebo and P. ginseng in improving anxiety. In view of the beneficial effect on the parameters assessed, the authors believe that this herbal medicine may represent, after larger studies, with larger samples and/or a higher dose of P. ginseng, a complementary form of therapy for fibromyalgia sufferers, or even in the event of a lack of response or the impossibility of carrying out conventional therapy (TRAN et al., 2021; PINTO-SANCHEZ ET al., 2021). According to some studies, this should be evaluated when advising patients on the use of complementary medicine, especially herbal medicines and dietary supplements. These include: natural medication is not always effective; many commercially available products do not guarantee efficacy and safety; the quantity and quality of active ingredients can vary from one product to another, and from one season to another in the same product; herbal products are not universally considered to be drugs and can be subject to contamination; the interaction of natural products with medicines in use by the patient can trigger serious consequences and, finally, the fact that some population groups such as children, pregnant women or women trying to conceive and the elderly should not receive any type of complementary medicine without medical supervision (FOGAÇA et al., 2021; SLYKERMAN et al., 2021).

REFERENCES

ABELES AM, PILLINGER MH, SOLITAR BM, ABELES M. Narrative review: the pathophysiology of fibromyalgia. Ann Intern Med. May 15, 2007;146(10):726-34. **Accessed on:** September 20, 2021.

BARBOSA, I., COSTA, I., BERNAL, M., & SOUZA, D. (2016). Rate trends mortality from the ten leading causes of cancer deaths in Brazil, 1996-2012. Rev. Ciênc. Plur, 2(1):3-16. **Accessed on:** September 20, 2021.

BARBOSA, K., COSTA, N., ALFENAS. R., PAULA. S., & MININ, V. (2010). Oxidative stress: concept, implications and modulating factors. Revista de Nutrição, v. 23, n. 4, p. 629-643. **Accessed on:** September 20, 2021.

BELLATO E, MARINI E, CASTOLDI F, BARBASETTI N, MATTEI L, BONASIA

DE, et al. Fibromyalgia Syndrome: Etiology, Pathogenesis, Diagnosis, and Treatment [Internet]. Pain Research and Treatment. 2012. Available at: https://www.hindawi.com/journals/prt/2012/426130/abs/. **Accessed on:** September 20, 2021.

BENNETT RM, FRIEND R, MARCUS D, BERNSTEIN C, HAN BK, YACHOUI R, et al. Criteria for the Diagnosis of Fibromyalgia: Validation of the Modified 2010 Preliminary American College of Rheumatology Criteria and the Development of Alternative Criteria. Arthritis Care Res. 1 de septiembre de 2014;66(9):1364-73. **Accessed on:** September 20, 2021.

CABEZAS SÁNCHEZ C, YAGUI MOSCOSO M, CABALLERO ÑOPO P, ESPINOZA SILVA M, CASTILLA T, GRANADOS A, et al. Prioridades de investigación en salud en el Perú2010-2014: la experiencia de un proceso participativo y descentralizado:sistematización de la experiencia [Internet]. Instituto Nacional de Salud; 2011. **Accessed on:** September 20, 2021.

CARABOTTI M, SCIROCCO A, MASELLI M A, SEVERIA C. The gut-brain axis: interactions between enteric microbiota, central and enteric nervous systems. Ann Gastroenterol. 2015 Apr-Jun; 28(2): 203-209. Available at < https://www.ncbi.nlm.nih.gov/pmc/articles/PMC4367209/>. **Accessed on:** September 20, 2021.

COHEN H. Controversies and challenges in fibromyalgia: a review and a proposal. Ther Adv Musculoskelet Dis. May 2017;9(5):115-27. **Accessed on:** September 20, 2021.

ESTÉVEZ-LÓPEZ F, SEGURA-JIMÉNEZ V, ÁLVAREZ-GALLARDO IC, BORGES-COSIC M, PULIDO-MARTOS M, CARBONELL-BAEZA A, et al. Adaptation profiles comprising objective and subjective measures in fibromyalgia: the al-Ándalus project. Rheumatol Oxf Engl. 1 de noviembre de 2017;56(11):2015-24. **Accessed on:** September 20, 2021.

FERRAN J. GARCIA. Blazing a trail. Basics of fibromyalgia, chronic fatigue and multiple chemical intolerance | Ferran j. Garcia | Comprar libro 9788496516113 [Internet]. [cited 2017 December 2]. Disponible en: https://www.casadellibro.com/libro-abriendo-camino-principios-basicos-de- fibromyalgia-fatiga-croni-ca-e-intoleracia-quimica-multiple/9788496516113/1108639. **Accessed on:** September 20, 2021.

FOGAÇA M V, DUMAN R S. Cortical GABAergic Dysfunction in Stress and Depression: New Insights for Therapeutic Interventions. Front Cell Neurosci. 2019;13:87.. https://doi.org/10.3389/fncel.2019.00087. **Accessed on:** Sep 20, 2021.

GAVANSKI, D., BARATTO, I., & GATTI, R. (2015). Evaluation of bowel habits and dietary fiber intake in an elderly population. Revista brasileira de obesidade, nutrição e emagrecimento, São Paulo. v.9. n.49. p.3-11. **Accessed on:** September 20, 2021.
GUMÀ-URIEL L, PEÑARRUBIA-MARÍA MT, CERDÀ-LAFONT M, CUNILLERA-PUERTOLAS O, ALMEDA-ORTEGA J, FERNÁNDEZ-VERGEL R, et al. Impact of IPDE-SQ personality disorders on the healthcare and societal costs of fibromyalgia patients: a cross-sectional study. BMC Fam Pract [Internet]. June 1, 2016 [cited 2017 December 6];17. Available at: https://www.ncbi.nlm.nih.gov/pmc/articles/PMC4888611/. **Accessed on:** September 20, 2021.

HOLZER P, FARZI A. Neuropeptides and the Microbiota-Gut-Brain Axis. Adv Exp Med Biol. 2014; 817: 195-219. https://doi.org/10.1007/978-1-4939-0897-4_9_ http://repositorio.ins.gob.pe/handle/INS/122.7. **Accessed on:** Sep 20, 2021.

LISETE H. Brain-derived neurotrophic factor in fibromyalgia syndrome. 2008. Available at <http://tede2.pucrs.br/tede2/bitstream/tede/5322/1/402410.pdf> Accessed on Mar 28, 2021. **Accessed on:** September 20, 2021.

LUNA R A, FOSTER J A. Gut brain axis: diet microbiota interactions and implications for modulation of anxiety and depression. Curr Opin Biotechnol. 2015 Apr;32:35-41. https://doi.org/10.1016/j.copbio.2014.10.007. **Accessed on:** September 20, 2021.

MORAES A L F, BUENO R G A L, FUENTES-ROJAS M, ANTUNES A E C.

Probiotic supplementation and depression: a therapeutic strategy? Rev. Ciênc. Méd., (Campinas). 2019;28(1): 31-47. **Accessed on:** September 20, 2021.

MÜLLER W, SCHNEIDER EM, STRATZ T. The classification of fibromyalgia syndrome. Rheumatol Int. septiembre 2007;27(11):1005-10. **Accessed on:** September 20, 2021.

OPIE R S, O'NEIL A, JACKA F N, PIZZINGA J, ITSIOPOULOS C. A modified Mediterranean dietary intervention for adults with major depression: dietary protocol and feasibility data from the smiles trial. Nutr Neurosci. 2018 Sep;21(7):487-501. https://doi.org/ 10.1080/1028415X.2017.1312841. **Accessed on:** September 20, 2021.

PASQUAL MARQUES, A. DE SOUSA DO ESPÍRITO SANTO, A. ASSUMPCAO BERSSANETI, L. AKEMI MATSUTANI, S. LEE KING YUAN. Prevalence of fibromyalgia: literature review update - ScienceDirect. Available at: http://www.sciencedirect.com/science/article/pii/S2255502117300056. **Accessed on:** September 20, 2021.

PERNAMBUCO AP, SILVA LRT DA, FONSECA ACS, REIS D'ÁVILA, PERNAMBUCO AP, SILVA LRT DA, et al. Clinical profile of patients with fibromyalgia syndrome. Fisioter Em Mov. April 2017;30(2):287-96. **Accessed on:** September 20, 2021.

PINTO-SANCHEZ M I, HALL G B, GHAJAR K, NARDELLI A, BOLINO C, LAU J T, et al. Probiotic bifidobacterium longum NCC3001 reduces depression scores and alters brain activity: A pilot study in patients with irritable bowel syndrome. Gastroenterology. 2017 Aug;153(2):448-459.e8. https://doi.org/10.1053/j.gastro.2017.05.003. **Accessed on:** September 20, 2021.

RIZZI M, RADOVANOVIC D, SANTUS P, AIROLDI A, FRASSANITO F, VANNI S, et al. Influence of autonomic nervous system dysfunction in the genesis of sleep disorders in fibromyalgia patients. Clin Exp Rheumatol. junio de 2017;35 Suppl

105(3):74-80. **Accessed on:** September 20, 2021.

RODRÍGUEZ A, TEMBL J, MESA-GRESA P, MUÑOZ MÁ, MONTOYA P, REY B. Altered cerebral blood flow velocity features in fibromyalgia patients in resting-state conditions. PloS One. 2017;12(7):e0180253. **Accessed on:** September 20, 2021.

SATOKARI, R., FUENTES, S., MATTILA, E., JALANKA, J., M. DE VOS, W., & ARKKILA, P. (2014). Fecal transplantation Treatment of antibiotic-induced noninfectious colitis and long-term microbiota monitoring. Case Reports in Medicine, New York, v. 2014, n. 913867, p. 1-7, nov. **Accessed:** Sep 20, 2021.

SLYKERMAN R F, HOOD F, WICKENS K, THOMPSON J M D, BARTHOW C, R MURPHY, KANG J, et al. Effect of Lactobacillus rhamnosus HN001 in Pregnancy on Postpartum Symptoms of Depression and Anxiety: A Randomized Double-blind Placebo-controlled Trial. EBioMedicine. 2017 Oct;24:159-165. https://doi.org/10.1016/j.ebiom.2017.09.013. **Accessed on:** September 20, 2021.

STILLING R M, DINAN T G, CRYAN J F. Microbial genes, brain & behavior - epigenetic regulation of the gut-brain axis. Genes Brain Behav. 2014 Jan;13(1):69-86. https://doi.org/10.1111/gbb.12109. **Accessed on:** Sep 20, 2021.

TOPRAK CELENAY, B. A. KULUNKOGLU, M. ERTUGRUL YASA, C. SAHBAZ PIRINCCI, U. NECMIYE YILDIRIM, O. KUCUKSAHIN, et al. A comparison of the effects of exercises plus connective tissue massage to exercises alone in women with fibromyalgia syndrome: a randomized contro... - PubMed - NCBI. Available at: https://www.ncbi.nlm.nih.gov/pubmed/28840379. **Accessed on:** September 20, 2021.

TRAN N, ZHEBRAK M, YACOUB C, PELLETIER J, HAWLEY D. The gut-brain relationship: Investigating the effect of multispecies probiotics on anxiety in a randomized placebo-controlled trial of healthy young adults. J Affect Disord. 2019 Jun 1;252:271-277. https://doi.org/10.1016/j.jad.2019.04.043. **Accessed on:** September 20, 2021.

ZHANG, Y., LI, S., GAN, R., ZHOU, T., XU, D., & LI, H. (2015). Impacts of intestinal bacteria in human health and disease. International Journal of Molecular Sciences. v.16, n.4, p.7493-7519. **Accessed on:** September 20, 2021.

CONTENTS

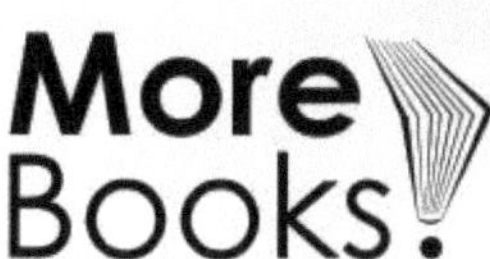

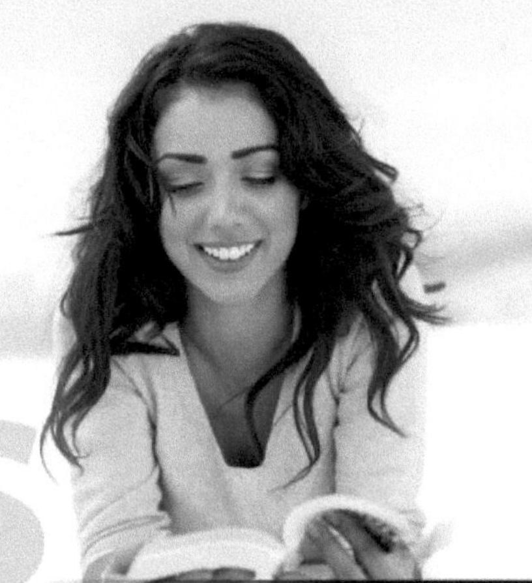

I want morebooks!

Buy your books fast and straightforward online - at one of world's fastest growing online book stores! Environmentally sound due to Print-on-Demand technologies.

Buy your books online at
www.morebooks.shop

Kaufen Sie Ihre Bücher schnell und unkompliziert online – auf einer der am schnellsten wachsenden Buchhandelsplattformen weltweit! Dank Print-On-Demand umwelt- und ressourcenschonend produzi ert.

Bücher schneller online kaufen
www.morebooks.shop

info@omniscriptum.com
www.omniscriptum.com

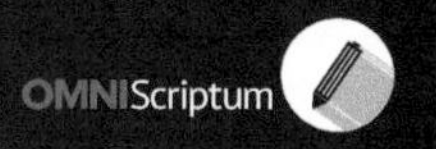

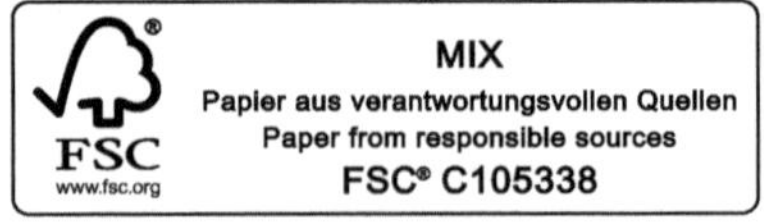

Printed by Books on Demand GmbH, Norderstedt / Germany